awakening fertility

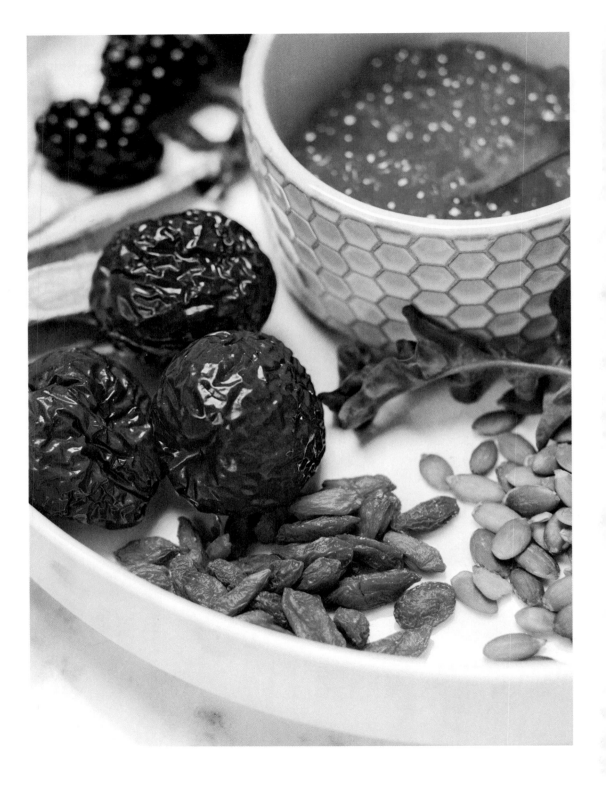

awakening fertility

*The Essential Art of
Preparing for Pregnancy*

HENG OU

AMELY GREEVEN AND MARISA BELGER

ABRAMS IMAGE, NEW YORK

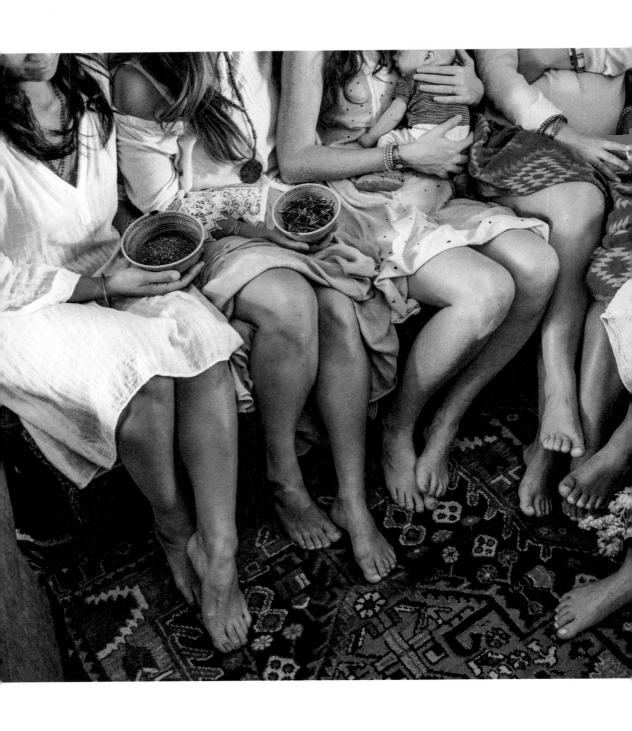

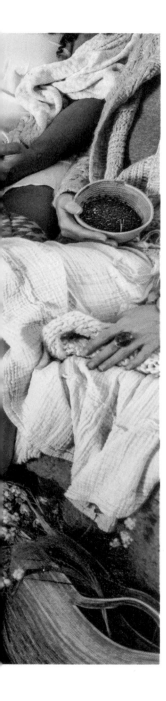

You want to have a baby.

The desire to become a mother, or a mother again, can manifest in many ways. It might bubble up out of the blue and surprise you, or it might pulse enduringly, like an ache that is never not felt. Whatever form it takes, the moment you feel this call toward childbearing, a doorway opens, leading you to a path that will take you from one version of yourself to the next. It is a path of becoming.

We take many journeys of becoming in our lives: becoming an adult; becoming a professional; becoming a partner or a spouse or a member of a community. Yet the path of becoming a mother is a phenomenon unto itself, one taken largely out of sight, as publicizing one's desire to conceive a child and the ups and downs involved still feels taboo to many. And it's one with a uniquely unfixed destination, in which pregnancy and motherhood can sometimes seem within easy reach and other times like a confounding, illusory mirage. You may be called toward having a baby, but when, how, and even if you'll arrive there are not factors you can predict or control.

What adds more layers of challenge is that, today, women tend to set out on their mission toward motherhood in something of a scramble, without proper briefing, backup, or help prepping and securing the vessel for safe, strong passage. All great voyagers know that a venture's success depends on deep preparation. Yet when it comes to pregnancy, we often take the leap without first strengthening our sea legs. It's not a stretch to say that many women today are highly stressed and minimally rested, overfed yet frequently also undernourished, and hyperconnected yet poorly supported.

Perhaps because pregnancy is such a clear and decisive state of being, full of excitement and possibility, it's easy to overlook, or even disregard, the more mundane preparation phase. But for a woman the consequences of skipping this phase are real, from having difficulty conceiving, to significant postpartum depletion (a baby takes what he or she needs in utero, even at the expense of the mother's well-being after birth), or simply experiencing a pervasive—and largely unnecessary!—anxiety about the whole process.

In traditional wellness practices, setting a course for pregnancy didn't leave a woman scrambling to make a lifestyle U-turn or abruptly dropping one way of being in order to take on another. Thanks to a continuum of self-care that was initiated when her fertility potential was first expressed—with the onset of menstruation—she was more ready and primed for conception when the time came. Early on, she was naturally guided into a lifestyle promoting inner balance and ongoing fortification, with the possibility of pregnancy always in mind. Today, our path toward pregnancy looks quite different—the women of yesteryear would no doubt be shocked at the way we embark on the journey toward motherhood! But how are we supposed to know better? Preparing for pregnancy is a conversation that isn't being had: this wisdom is not passed down from mother to daughter, is not shared in school, and it's not a topic that your doctor will bring up. As a society, we like results but get bored with process; we love to gaze at destinations but don't have the patience to hear about the journey. Making space for all that occurs along the intimate path to becoming a mother, and finding support during the bumps on the road, can be a challenge—if we're even aware that this preparation time is something we deserve to claim for ourselves!

Reclaiming these vital phases of the mothering journey and supporting a woman—not just her baby—through every stage is my focus and my passion. Ten years ago, I began cooking food for new mothers inspired by the traditions of postpartum care and nourishment I had inherited from the Chinese medicine healers in my Chinese-American family. I called my food-delivery service MotherBees, to help each new woman feel like part of a buzzing hive of care at a time when she can so often feel alone. The idea struck a chord—turns out there was quite a need for this kind of care!—and I recruited two good friends, the writers Amely Greeven and Marisa Belger, to create a book called *The First Forty Days*. It translated the traditional Chinese protocols of *zuo yuezi*, or confinement care, into something more fit for modern families' lives—replete with comforting and rebuilding recipes.

The First Forty Days shone a spotlight on a long overlooked phase of the mothering journey—the early days and weeks after the birth of a baby—and reminded us collectively to honor the needs of a woman in this time. In weaving together global postpartum protocols, we discovered just how much targeted care for the new mother influences recovery, bonding, and replenishment, and carries longer-term consequences for her health and well-being. Inspired, we invited women and their partners to learn these principles before giving birth and to reframe the early weeks after delivering their baby as a sacred period of rest and recovery instead of viewing it as a trampoline to launch them back to an earlier version of themselves.

The response to *The First Forty Days* took our breath away, as one woman shared it with another, often posting pictures on social media of the book open on her kitchen counter or in a stack of night-table reads preparing her for what's to come. Midwives, doulas, and obstetricians began telling us they were giving the book to pregnant clients as a way to extend their reach of maternal care past the baby's arrival. To this day, we receive messages from women around the world sharing how they are making space for a supported first forty days—and underneath the images of the homemade soups and stews they're preparing before birth or receiving during their recovery is a sense of relief: *I'm not the only one going through this moody, sweaty, unpredictable phase of adjustment and upheaval. Someone else really gets it. I'm not alone.*

A couple of years after the publication of *The First Forty Days*, women began asking us a whole new kind of question: Was there a *zuo yuezi*–like protocol of food and self-care they could use *before* becoming pregnant, to help conception come more easily and pregnancy go smoothly? The truth is, there was not. In the old, traditional ways of Chinese medicine, from an early age women were guided to care for their "essence of life," called *jing*, to regulate their menstrual cycle, and to eat earthy, building, and restorative whole foods that nourished their reproductive center in anticipation of their mothering years. It was an ongoing lifestyle of caring for fertility potential, not a short program. Could we shake this out, we wondered, extract the essential nuggets from this continuum of self-care and turn them into something modern women could use? It had never been done before.

And so this book was conceived.

We began a wide-ranging exploration of the subject, each one of us putting out the call to our circles of practitioners, healers, guides, and mentors—the wise women and wise men, too, who have generously brought their profound depths of experience and wisdom to our mothering books (see page 16 for a full list). In *The First Forty Days*, we shared how Chinese medicine sees the womb as the "baby room," and how *after* birth, we must take great care of that room to ensure it doesn't get exposed to disruptive forces that can significantly affect a woman's well-being for months and years to come. Now we wanted to know, how could a woman (and her mate if she has one) build and furnish that baby room considerably *before* pregnancy? Going deeper still, how could she prepare her *whole* self for the monumental changes that conceiving a child involves— her body, her mind, and her spirit?

As mothers, our first point of research is always ourselves. I had grown up steeped in the traditional protocols of my Chinese-healer ancestors, been served special foods and herbs at different phases of my menstrual cycle, been chided to wear socks to keep my reproductive center warm (energy channels that support it start in the feet), and been encouraged to feed all kinds of virility-boosting foods to my partner before conceiving our children. Amely, meanwhile, had followed the nutrient-dense eating protocols of Weston A. Price—wild game, raw milk, and liver—on the advice of her Viking-like chiropractor and performed hormone-balancing liver cleanses in the lead-up to becoming a mother. Marisa had cleansed and prepared in her own way, actively connecting to the spirit of her first baby and surrendering to the unexpected conception of her second— processes that established the groundwork for peaceful and resilient parenting. Healthy lifestyles are our own geeky passions—this stuff is what we consider fun! We wondered if the easeful conceptions and robust babies that resulted were proof that early preconception preparation really does pay off.

The wise ones said yes. And everything else they shared—the knowledge you will discover in the chapters that follow—only stoked our passion for pregnancy preparation further. There are so many layers to this subject, and it's said that when you ask for teachers, they appear. In our case, we connected with Ayurvedic doctors from India; mystical healers and meditation teachers from

Europe; herbal alchemists and trauma facilitators from the Americas; Chinese medicine doctors from Australia; and my own family of acupuncturists. One person led us to the next, and a circle of experts formed around us—a village of sorts, luminaries standing ready with torches lit, offering to help make the journey toward mothering more supported. (What a gift, in an age where it's so easy to get lost in internet wormholes, looking for answers about all things maternity in a sea of confusing chatter!)

Their combined wisdom had never been gathered and woven together into one book. As we did the wordsmithing, their thoughts confirmed what we already knew to be true: that preparing to become a mother doesn't stop at the physical aspects of our being. While nutritious and uncontaminated food, good sleep, exercise, and a toxic-free environment are essential, they fall flat without the counterbalance of a clear and open heart, active and trusted intuition, and consistent bursts of joy. These more esoteric aspects team up with vital physical health to form a truly fertile life, the ideal backdrop for the unpredictable road to motherhood.

Of course, let's not forget the cooking part! I will always put eating at the center of all self-care. But not just for the obvious reasons. For me, food has multidimensional influence. Yes, food builds your reserve of important nutrients for conception, pregnancy, and healthy fetal development. To that end, the forty-six recipes in this book are designed to provide a well-rounded approach to pre-conception nourishment and are replete with the vitamins, minerals, proteins, fats, and protective compounds that mother, father, and child require, free of the additives and stimulants that can have such disruptive effect, and accented with ingredients that the old ways knew could help create conditions for conception and pregnancy. My hope is that using them not only makes wholesome eating easier, but that it piques your curiosity about all the ways food can make you feel stronger, clearer, more ready for what's ahead, and most of all, more connected to your body. But it's also even simpler than that. Food is also love, the doorway into caring daily for yourself. Cooking is in some ways the heart of this book, because I believe it can be the way you start to mother yourself and your partner,* setting yourself up for a healthy experience of mothering a child.

Like *The First Forty Days*, this is not a typical cookbook. The recipes are surrounded by gestures of guidance and insights for inspiration. You'll find meditation practices, ways of tapping into the powerful energy of the womb, and gentle methods of releasing mental and emotional blocks that may be tripping you up as you move forward. Each one is an ingredient that you can place in your self-care pot, to feed you in this process of becoming. Consider this a book full of recipes for eating *and* for being and living—each designed to support and sustain you in all the ways women really need when inviting in this dynamic new phase of life. Some of this guidance may seem a little out-there. Stay with us! To address the full person, we want always to look at how the mind, body, and spirit are doing, and to illuminate all the layers of possibility that come into play— even the ones hiding in the corner that we tend not to talk about.

Like anything of meaning, preparing consciously for pregnancy requires some effort and even some letting go of your current or preferred ways of doing things—whether that's burning the candle at both ends with too much work or play, skipping balanced meals, or indulging in frequent caffeine boosts or boozy escapades. But this giving up of one way of doing things will serve you in the near and far future; you are strengthening a key muscle that you will use endlessly in motherhood and in any other venture in life. Motherhood asks you to be relentlessly selfless, to give up ways of being that you've held on to for decades, even for always. The principles of balance and fortification in these pages will serve you at every stage of your life. They are as much my bedrocks today with teenagers in the house as they were before those teens were twinkles in their parents' eyes.

In Chinese medicine, the philosophy of health and longevity is rooted in the idea of a healthy garden. Our role is to tend to the earth of our well-being in a daily way, with the care and compassion of a devoted gardener. We must pay attention to the soil, nourishing and feeding it, and to the quality of the water, anticipate changes in weather and protect what we're growing from one

* A quick note here: In this book we most often refer to a woman's partner or mate in the masculine for the simplicity of writing, but our intention is inclusive; if your family looks different, we hope you can see yourselves in our words.

season to the next. This means we want to start tending our soil as early as possible if we hope to plant a seed and grow new life. The best soil has had years of thoughtful TLC before taking on even one seed.

As you may have guessed by now, this book is not intended to be a guide to solving fertility issues that may have taken some time to manifest. Our focus here is to help you establish fertility-protecting habits early on, ideally before actively moving toward pregnancy, and ideally *before* challenges show up. "Fertility protecting," you ask? Yes. As you will discover, fertility is not something to be boosted or manipulated. It is a potential that we can protect and preserve—even as we age—and also recover if it's gone into hiding, which can very often be due to lifestyle-related causes. It's important to note that recovering this potential is typically a task in which years of clinical practice comes in handy. The principles in this book may well help you regulate your menstrual cycle (and learn a bit about your ovulation dates), which on its own can have powerful positive effects. However, if you are currently experiencing chronic issues that seem to be hampering your dreams of pregnancy—such as PCOS, endometriosis, miscarriage, or any other imbalance—I recommend enlisting the guidance of a trusted and well-reviewed Chinese medicine practitioner or another expert practitioner of your choice, and then leaning on all the insights in this book simultaneously.

By making a commitment to prepare for pregnancy, you are joining a growing population of women who are tapping into a desire to understand and care for their bodies more deeply. As we become increasingly aware that we are living in an age of lower levels of nutrition and higher levels of toxicity—and anxiety—there is a new surge of interest in fertility awareness and prenatal health. More and more resources in this arena are appearing in the form of prenatal diet books, fertility-tracking apps, women's wellness and spiritual groups, and impassioned health and lifestyle bloggers. And, as new understanding of the science of epigenetics solidifies, some terrific teachers are sharing how our lifestyle choices today influence not only the well-being of our unborn children, but *their* children, too. This is all contributing to a heightened awareness of how each decision we make, even the really small ones, can have a powerful trickle-down effect, and how much power we actually have to create conditions for a happier, healthier life.

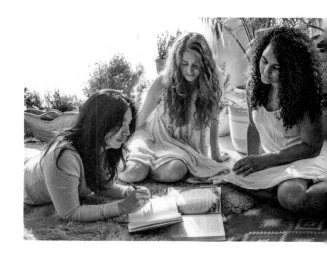

Yet a strange hushed tone still wraps itself around the process of conceiving a child. You can shout it from the rooftops when it happens, with clever Facebook posts, family dinner announcements, and "gender reveal" parties, but isn't it odd that along the way there wasn't any room to talk about the twists and turns that occurred or to share the experiences you learned from or would do differently next time? When the thoughts, feelings, and experiences surrounding a process that is primal and part of all of us—whether we want to procreate or not—are cloaked in secrecy, it can lead to shame and even trauma. We see this urge to forge a new way reflected in the women warriors who are courageous enough to be open about a miscarriage or fertility treatment, who refuse to let confounding health issues or even a hysterectomy get in the way of their dream, or who break the rules and announce a pregnancy before the three-month norm, daring their friends and family to remain steady if there is a complication. Because sometimes there is a complication. These pioneers remind us that there are so many women who sit in painful silence. It's time the subject of becoming a mother—the entire subject, with its many layers and nuances—was out in the open. With *The First Forty Days*, we witnessed the power of women circling up to share their experiences, their truths—and their recipes, too—taking the postpartum phase out of the shadows and holding it up as something necessary and good. Now let's shine the light on the pre-pregnancy conversation, talking about the process before it gets hard, so we can lean on and learn from each other—making our march toward motherhood something that brings us together as women, and as a society at large.

THE WISE ONES

Much of the wisdom shared in *Awakening Fertility* was born from conversations with the following experts, who graciously gave their time and energy to supporting this project. We could not have written this book without their thoughtful guidance.

ELLIANA ALLON and **ALISON RITCHIE,** founders of Of Oaks and Owls, a women's wellness movement focusing on birth and postpartum services, Winnipeg, Canada *www.instagram.com/ofoaksandowls*

KATHERINE ALEXANDER ANDERSON, doctor of acupuncture and Chinese medicine, founder and clinical director of Rhythms, an integrative healthcare and acupuncture clinic with holistic fertility services, Portland, Maine *www.rhythmsforwomen.com*

JULIA BAROKOV, LMFT, spiritual psychotherapist, Oakland, California *www.juliabarokov.com*

BRIANNA BATTLES, MS, CSCS, founder of Pregnancy and Postpartum Athleticism, Thousand Oaks, California *www.briannabattles.com*

CHAD CORNELL, master herbalist and holistic therapist, Winnipeg, Canada *www.hollowreedholistic.ca*

LAUREN CURTAIN, women's health acupuncturist and Chinese medicine practitioner, Victoria, Australia *www.laurencurtain.com*

NORA GEDGAUDAS, CNS, NTP, BCHN, author, clinician, educator, ketogenically-based ancestral nutrition expert, Portland, Oregon *www.primalbody-primalmind.com*

LACEY HAYNES, founder of School of Whole and creator of Pussy Gazing, London, United Kingdom *www.laceyhaynes.com*

JAPA KHALSA, doctor of Oriental medicine and certified yoga therapist C-IAYT, coauthor of the book *Enlightened Bodies*, Española, New Mexico *www.drjapa.com*

LINDA LANCASTER, ND, founder of Light Harmonics Institute, Santa Fe, New Mexico *www.lightharmonics.com*

JILLIAN LAVENDER, Vedic wellness expert, cofounder of New York Meditation Center and London Meditation Centre, London, United Kingdom *www.vedicmeditation.net*

IN SOOK LEE, LAc, doctor of acupuncture specializing in women's hormones, digestion, and fertility, Burbank, California

JAY LOKHANDE, MD, MBA in biotechnology, doctor of Ayurveda, and expert in formulating botanical and biotech drug products, Los Angeles, California
www.indusextracts.com

MARCIA LOPEZ, holistic reproductive wellness practitioner, owner of Women's True Healing, Redondo Beach, California
www.womenstruehealing.com

PAULA MALLIS, doula, founder of WMN Space, Culver City, California
www.wmnspace.com

KAREN PAUL, holistic nutritionist, The Source Natural Foods, Kailua, Hawaii
www.thesourcenatural.com

TIBBY PLASSE, real food advocate, writer, and development director for Flourish Foundation, Victor, Idaho
www.flourishfoundation.com

ULRIKE REMLEIN, womb awakening mentor and red tent facilitator, Regensburg, Germany
www.wombofjoy.com

ALISON SINATRA, women's circle facilitator, yoga instructor, High Falls, New York
www.alloursacredsisters.com
www.alisonsinatra.net

DANICA THORNBERRY, LAc, doctor of acupuncture and Oriental medicine, specializing in women's reproductive health, founder of the Seed Fertility Program, Los Angeles, California
www.wellwomenacupuncture.com
www.seedfertility.com

V. A. VENUGOPAL, MD, founder of Ashtangavaidyam Ayurvedics, Kerala, India, and Ayurvedic mentor at HANAH
www.ayurvedakerala.com
www.hanahlife.com

SARAH VILLAFRANCO, MD, founder of Osmia Organics, Carbondale, Colorado
www.osmiaorganics.com

NEESHA ZOLLINGER, Anusara yoga instructor, founder of Akasha Yoga, Jackson, Wyoming
www.neeshazollingeryoga.com

AND MY RELATIONS:

JU CHUN OU, aka Auntie Ou, Chinese medicine practitioner and acupuncturist, Oakland, California

CHING CHUN OU, Chinese medicine practitioner, acupuncturist, and fertility expert, Oakland, California

LI-CHUN OU, Chinese medicine practitioner and herbalist, Oakland, California

1

the three universal themes and the five realms of discovery

My fascination with making babies began early. In one of my earliest memories, I'm roving the hallways of my relatives' Chinese medicine offices in Oakland, California, catching fragments of conversation from behind closed doors. I hear my Auntie Ou, an herbalist renowned for her expertise in reproductive health, describing in her uniquely choppy English what must be in place for "catching the egg." She says that this feat successfully occurs "if eggs come on time, if sperm is good, if both parents truly desire a child, and if the baby room is ready."

C atching the egg? Readying a baby room? My eight-year-old imagination took flight, picturing luminescent ova dropping from the skies, landing with a *poof!* in a cushy, inviting haven. As I got older, I understood that she was helping couples create the optimal conditions for becoming parents. Auntie Ou, who at seventy-six is semi-retired, with a golf-putting mat in her office, is not the sentimental type. She delivers her advice at a rapid clip and doesn't do chitchat, but she's passionate about preparing a woman and her mate for the life-changing act of conceiving, carrying, and delivering a child. According to her healing lineage, proper preconception care not only helps pregnancy come more easily; it ensures mom is stronger during and after the forty weeks of gestation, throughout her mothering days, and into menopause. Very importantly, it also creates a robust offspring replete with the health, longevity, and—vain as this sounds—attractive looks that come when parents-to-be are chock-full of essential nutrients and filled to brimming with the "essence of life" called jing. It's a generational thing: every elder wants to see their family line carried forward on the wings of brains, beauty, and just a touch of brawn—the total package!

I also heard anxious voices behind the closed doors and, sometimes, the sound of crying. Often, new patients came because they were experiencing struggles on their journey to conceive. This didn't faze Auntie Ou, or her acupressurist sister, or her herbalist brother, who both would help treat patients as needed; she didn't believe in the concept of infertility. Auntie is expert at diagnosing the imbalances that occur when our systems are under stress or not getting the support they require that can affect fertility in both partners.

She knows these patterns show up differently in each person; her job is to follow the patterns back to their root cause, then address them with diet, herbs and acupuncture, and even mind-body practices to move the vital energy or *chi*. Brushing off excessive concerns about "advanced maternal age" or previous reproductive problems, she likes to say, "When a woman's body is in balance and harmony, then she will bear fruit." (Ditto, in her books, for the man, who quite often needs help for his "sluggish" or "sleepy" sperm.) I recall how she'd have her couples return to her clinic weekly for some months, as she would reliably nudge their bodies out of any slump so they could rise into their parenting potential. "We're waking up mom and dad," I once heard her say, as if the mother- and father-to-be had just been napping for a while.

Of course, the intricacies of procreation were still a mystery to me. But this early education set in my mind that motherhood was not something that just happened to you—"Surprise! We're expecting!" It happened through a gradual dawning, a slow and steady season of preparation and self-care. It also sparked my wonder for the unseen ecosystem in which babies are made and born, and an enthrallment with this hidden place of power that I then didn't quite understand but explored through my art. My preteen sketchbooks are filled with charcoal drawings of curving fallopian tubes and watercolors of plush, pink uteruses, and sometimes a tiny egg making its incredible voyage to—if it was its lucky day!—meet its destined sperm. This was several decades before today's rebirth of heightened menstrual awareness, lunar-phase Instagram posts, and apps and technology for ovulation tracking. My dreamy Piscean womb doodles, had anyone glimpsed them, would have been thought quite strange.

When the time came for my first menstrual cycle, then, I had a foot in both worlds. I felt just as awkward and uncomfortable with the rite of passage as any other American girl (and maybe more so, for my circumstances were such that I didn't have a nurturing maternal figure or older sisters at home), but simultaneously quite connected to my period as a focal point of health. I'd picked up enough from my aunties to know that premenstrual symptoms, changes in blood flow, and irregularities in cycle length were mirrors reflecting my broader state of health, because everything in the body is connected. Auntie

Ou would describe the different systems as interconnecting, like freeways that meet at interchanges, cars moving from one to the next. Like all my friends, I had moments of deep embarrassment and even shame around my monthly bleeding, wrapping a sweatshirt around my waist at school to hide the fact I'd been taken by surprise and awkwardly stashing pads and tampons in my cart at the supermarket. But as I moved beyond adolescence and into my twenties, I developed an awe for my four-week cycle. Here was my monthly report card, telling me if I was burning the candle at both ends, or if I'd been eating too many foods my digestion couldn't handle, or even if I was burying anger or ignoring stress. Rather than being an inconvenience—or, as previous generations called it, a curse—my period, and my whole cycle, was my gateway into knowing my body better. I learned to drink hot water in the days before my period to avoid "sticky blood" and stir the iron-rich herb dong quai into my soup as a blood builder afterward. As I got older and had more means, I tweaked my diet and lifestyle when the report card hinted that my Liver* *chi* was stagnant, and a migraine might start—acupuncture helped with that—or my Kidney energy was weak, and I needed to eat a moderate piece of high-quality steak. And—voilà!—I morphed from the girl who sketched reproductive systems in her notebooks into the young woman who could talk at length about the health implications of the color and viscosity of menstrual blood! I'm grateful for this now. This grandmotherly wisdom helped me understand that women's bodies are always in ebb and flow, and that we can gracefully ride the changing waves with adjustments in food, and rest, and supplemental herbs. If we listen, we can ward off depletions or imbalances early. It helped me develop an open dialogue with my body that it takes many women years to develop.

It wasn't until I was close to thirty that the awe for my body's creative power became truly personal. That's when I began to feel the stirring of my own awakening fertility—I wanted to have a baby! Looking back, I understand how my peripatetic lifestyle, fueled by wanderlust and foodie curiosity, had set me up well. I was living in Europe with my then partner, and I loved shopping

---

* A note: In this book, the traditional Chinese medicine (TCM) organ systems are capitalized, while the use actual anatomical organs are lowercase.

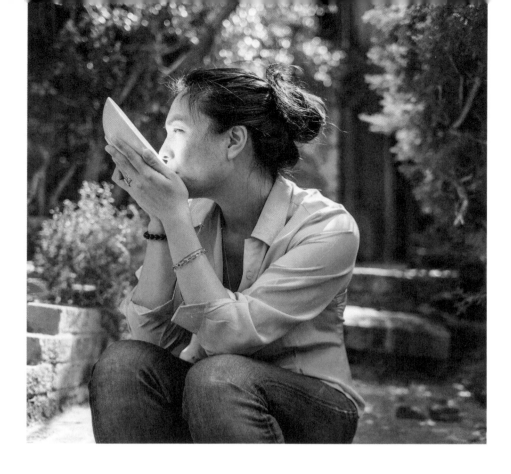

at traditional butchers and waterfront fish stands; I reveled in trying old-timey dishes using the weird stuff like offal or marrow that until quite recently were considered very uncool. I made broth galore from vegetables and bones—it's a custom in Chinese households to drink broth daily to help digestion—and I never passed a farm stand groaning with fresh vegetables or vibrant summer fruits without stopping. As it turned out, many of these fortifying foods nourish Kidney jing—the epicenter of reproductive force, according to Chinese medicine—as well as confer the nutrients that help the Liver and Spleen systems digest food well, build the blood, and provide the building material for hormones, all things that even from a more Western mind-set are also seen as pivotal for healthy pregnancy. My Chinese family might not have loved that I was living far from home, roaming English highways and byways, but they clucked approvingly at the fortifying diet of shellfish, steak-and-kidney pie, and heaps of watercress and spinach that I was consuming. "Now play music every day and relax!" came one missive from Auntie Ou, offering the next piece of the baby-making puzzle. "No thoughts for anything less than happiness." Her parting shot for me and my partner: "No every day together." Now that we had laid the physical groundwork, she advised we practice some restraint in lovemaking, or the sperm and the baby room—which I now understood to be her term for my uterus—and our hopeful state of mind would get too strained and tired.

I'll never know how much this preparation paved the way for the fluid experience of my first conception and, with time, the two pregnancies that followed. I feel blessed beyond measure that this part of the mothering story came easily. I do know that in each case, the connection I'd been fortunate to develop with my body helped me intuit exactly when I was ready to conceive, as if feeling an inner whisper. To this day, I can feel the alchemy of practical knowledge and ancestral wisdom that surrounded me in those years. Did eating fresh oysters galore with my partner in Auntie Ou's leafy, airy kitchen and learning her time-honored methods for conceiving a boy manifest our third beautiful child, Jude? (For the curious, it's three orgasms in the woman first, to balance acid levels in her vagina, then her turning onto her left side after her mate ejaculates, versus onto her right side for a girl.) Was it the clear intention and hazy dreams that helped, the active imagining of each child? Or was it sheer biology—the outcome of good timing and great nutrition? What I know for sure is that my lifestyle had made me attuned to my ovulation window and my menstrual cycle regular; I felt rejuvenated and ready, thanks to my repository of rest, and well fed and fortified, thanks to my eating habits.

Mine is quite a different scenario from the experiences I came to hear about as, after Jude's birth, I began to participate professionally in the birthing world, cooking food for new moms. Stories from the wise healers and doctors I met reinforced the split perspectives I'd experienced; one new friend, the Chinese medicine doctor Katherine Alexander Anderson, described her time working in hospitals in China. "Girls would come for help with menstrual irregularities in their late teens and were already recording their basal body temperatures to track their cycles—not to get pregnant, but because they knew their menstrual cycles are the bedrock of their fertility." Katherine contrasted this with her practice in Portland, Maine. "Only a very few patients come to *prepare* for fertility; most come only after struggling for years."

Her tale struck a chord. The prevailing mind-set of American culture is that a woman—and her partner—should be able to jump into pregnancy from a standing stop, when she decides it's time. All too often for a super-busy, already pressed-to-the-max modern woman, pre-pregnancy health is a "when/then" scenario, as in, "When I get pregnant, *then* I'll eat like a wellness warrior, clean up my lifestyle, and get serious about sleep." She might invest plenty of thinking—or stressing—into the project of starting a family, but the longer-term self-care that could help her get to that outcome can be an afterthought. (For that matter, even learning the basic knowledge of exactly when in her cycle she can become pregnant can be an afterthought, too!)

Or the other extreme might play out: type-A anxiety to get everything about fertility and pregnancy absolutely on point and totally under control. Late-night scrolling—alone and bleary-eyed after a long day of work—for nuggets of data to perfect the quest for conception. *How long should it take? Have I consumed the exact proportion of wild-caught* everything *and (super-expensive!) superfoods to build the perfect human? Wait, this is taking a while—do I need intervention, experts, and treatments?* Even for nonperfectionists, there is a paradox at play. Conceiving a child involves the ability to surrender and receive—the nervous system needs to feel soothed, settled, and safe to divert energetic resources to reproduction. Yet everyday life demands that women constantly do more, be more, and produce more; stopping to surrender to their body's quiet rhythms and deep, unspoken needs is not part of the game. America in the twenty-first century is all about polarity; when it comes to our bodies and our children, it can be hard to place our feet on middle ground.

The more I cooked for mothers, the more I could detect the psychic temperature around our modern maternal conundrum; the process of becoming pregnant was making a lot of women unsettled or even anxious. And anxiety about conception begets fatigue; then more fatigue creates more anxiety; and all of this makes that fruit-bearing state of "balance and harmony" feel so

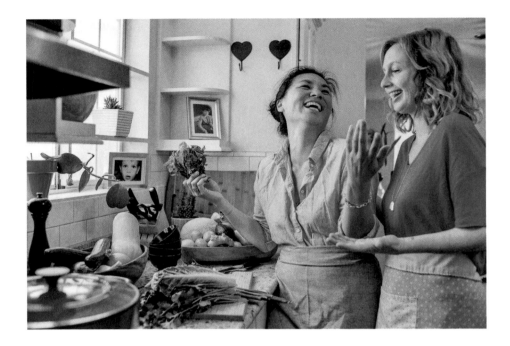

much further away. It was no wonder that so many women wrapped the journey toward pregnancy in words like "trying" and "struggle," yet barely had a conversation about it until they were on the other side. It was as if we were all walking to the edge of the diving board blindfolded, half expecting it'd be simple to whip off the eye mask and do a swan dive into pregnancy—and half fearful that we'd flail, or need expensive medical help along the way, yet unsure who to turn to in order to feel more grounded or secure. And so my inner circle—my cowriters, Marisa and Amely—and I began asking how it could be different. What if we started the conversation about pregnancy sooner, and leaned into the lifestyle that supports a mother-to-be in her quest a lot earlier? What if we pooled the older knowledge that our elders held about preparing for pregnancy with the new understandings of the pressures of this time, and then held each other in confidence and trust as we explored it together? It seemed to us that this might allow the mother within us to stir and awaken at a more reasonable pace, then take gradual, unhurried steps toward her destination, rather than leap up with a start, feeling foggy-headed, pressured, and already late.

When we started asking elders and wisdom keepers about the ways in which women had traditionally prepared for pregnancy, we knew enough to know there wouldn't be a single formula or protocol that fit every woman's needs for creating and sustaining balance. After all, each person has different physical and mental tendencies and constitutions; different health histories, life circumstances, and current health challenges. Medicines of all traditions have typically tailored approaches to the individual in question, subtly adjusting imbalances. But what, we wondered, would the *general* guidelines be, those that supported most people most of the time, laid the foundation for deeper inquiry if it were warranted, and let us layer new considerations for our modern era, as needed, on top?

It should be said upfront: I'm not a clinician; I'm a chef, mother, business owner, and champion of mothers, fathers, and families who supports them through the picture-perfect parts of parenting, and the messy moments, too, by nourishing them, body and soul. Addressing deeply entrenched fertility issues is not in my wheelhouse. Yet as we initiated conversations around preconception care with our wise ones—the practitioners, healers, mentors, and guides we turn to for help in our own lives and to inspire our maternal wellness books—a common theme arose. So often, women end up facing fertility challenges because our bodies have fallen out of balance long before we even contemplated motherhood, but we never addressed the instability. Putting awareness on our fertility potential at an earlier age can help lessen the chances of challenges arising later; while a woman and her partner may need expert help or intervention at some point along the path, if she's been living for years with at least one eye on balance and harmony, she'll likely end up requiring a lot less than she might think.

You're not only preparing for the conception of a child; you're preparing to give birth to your own higher selves.

—CHAD CORNELL, master herbalist and holistic therapist

We turned first to the indigenous traditions of the Northern Americas. The medicine wheel, a sacred tool marked with the four directions used in healing and ceremony, teaches us that everything in life is connected and cyclical. When it comes to understanding our passage into parenthood, these cultures view east as representing preconception, for in the east is where the sun rises; where new beginnings start and new days dawn. These cultures have long taught that there is a phase of life between adolescence and true adulthood that involves preparing for creating new life, in which a young woman and man take care of themselves in anticipation of becoming parents. That care—like the medicine wheel itself—encompasses the spiritual, mental, emotional, *and* physical dimensions of oneself.

Next, we learned from the Central and Southern Americas. In Southern California, Marcia Lopez, a women's wellness practitioner of Guatemalan ancestry, shared how techniques of *sobada*, or abdominal massage, have been used to tend to reproductive health at all stages of a woman's fertile life. This hands-on practice releases tension, promotes circulation of blood and energy so stagnation doesn't build up, and strengthens or even repositions the uterus if tension patterns have caused misalignment. As blood flows into every nook and cranny where stress, a sedentary lifestyle, or even trauma has previously blocked its freest flow, the woman's eggs receive more oxygen, helping to preserve their vitality. And the careful manual adjustments help to switch on the nervous system's calm state of functioning, which can help to restore overall hormonal balance and thereby address menstrual irregularity or discomfort around the cycle.

From Korea, we learned by talking to dear friends how wannabe moms were chided by their grandmas for sitting on the floor, a pillow always swiftly inserted under descending bottoms. Cold, the elders warned, would impede circulation and warmth, both requisites for reproductive balance. Meanwhile, served on a woman's daily plate were foods that resemble ovarian sacs, such as orange segments and pomegranate seeds. In Korea, as in many cultures that still take wisdom from old medicines, a food is more than just its nutritional components; its look, taste, smell, texture, and shape all communicate messages to the body, switching on certain functions just the way enzymes or probiotics do. (Thus, an ovary-like food encourages healthy ova in us; the same is true in Ayurveda, which prizes black sesame seeds for that reason.) Our reporting Korean-American granddaughter shared the succinct edict given by her wizened herbalist: *Yin her up!* Like many women who, say, actually have to make a living and provide for themselves in a rat race, she'd tipped to an extreme in which her natural yin—the slower, quieter, yet sustaining aspect of nature—energy had become overly dominated by yang, the highly active and generative aspect.

When we turned to Ayurveda, the "science of life" that originates in the Vedic knowledge of ancient India and dates back five thousand years (it's so old, it's said to be the origin of traditional Chinese medicine!), we discovered it offered a structured philosophy about preparing for pregnancy, so ingrained in the tradition that its preparation guidelines are actually taught to Ayurvedic doctors in training. Its precepts teach that both mother- and father-to-be are to deliberately care for four fundamental needs, getting them all in place. The first is rtu, the "season" chosen for pregnancy. Planning the right time includes personally, in terms of a woman's fertility; globally, in terms of peace and well-being in the world, and even cosmically, with the stars aligning for astrological benevolence. The second is *kshetra*, the "field" in which the baby will grow; this refers to having a healthy womb, the mother's body being free of *ama*, or a toxic buildup of material the body preferably should excrete, as well as having a balance of the three *doshas*, or energies of the body, and a regular menstrual cycle. The third is *ambu*, the "waters" that bring life to the field; mother and father should ensure that all the fluids and natural chemicals that circulate in the parents' bodies—blood, plasma, lymph, and hormones, as well as foods and water—are in peak condition. And the fourth is *bija*, the highest-quality "seed" of the egg and the sperm, which is not only determined by the quality of food, but by the quality of *everything* the parents digest, including thoughts, feelings, and experiences, which all have an impact and may skew positive or negative. (This influence can be especially meaningful for the male, who is generating new "seeds" on a bi- to tri-monthly basis.) In Ayurveda, bija is one expression of *ojas*, the super-subtle, most refined life-giving substance in the body that is the ultimate product of digestion, made thirty days after food is consumed. Ojas is responsible not just for the potency of fertility, but for the glow of luminous skin, the strength of immunity, the grace of aging, the clarity of a strong mind, and even the physical manifestation of a conscious spirit—in a sense, it is the numinous glow of life.

Think of Ayurveda's systematic approach to preconception like a gardener's guide to preparing for fruitful harvest: it helps her pick the right season for planting, then build healthy soil; it helps her water the terrain with clean water and enrich it with amendments. Then it encourages her to plant the best seeds she can, with deliberation and patience. All the while, a woman is being guided in six other, less tangible areas, relating to the *way* she and her mate prepare for pregnancy—around achieving a higher state of consciousness; around developing the strength of mind to live disciplined lifestyles, especially in eating, sleeping, and sexual activity; and ultimately, around bringing connection and sacredness to the act of conception itself.

It's impossible to look into global preconception care without exploring the work of Weston A. Price, the dentist who in the 1930s performed pioneering research on the ways industrialized foods disrupt the body's natural patterns of growth and development. For years, he traveled around the globe to study societies who followed indigenous lifestyles and ate traditional foods from their immediate environment without any processing, refining, or industrial methods of production. One of his most notable insights was that cultures in every part of the world saved the most nutritious foods—those with the greatest volume of vitamins, minerals, and, especially, precious fatty acids—for parents-to-be, pregnant women, and breastfeeding mothers, and also for children, knowing how profoundly they fed into a child's physical and mental development. As refined foods and sugars from the industrialized food system found their ways into traditional diets, Price observed radical declines in the skeletal and soft tissue development of offspring, as well as in their general health, resiliency, and temperament. He also noted how many societies endorsed spacing pregnancies three years apart, to make sure mothers had time to fortify themselves before their next conception.

Our findings about preconception protocols were not limited to physical and mental robustness, however. Some of the wisdom-keepers we spoke with put the greatest emphasis *not* on what a parent-to-be should eat or drink, but rather on the higher state of awareness they could achieve as they entered this phase of life and the sacredness of procreation. From Kerala, India, the renowned Ayurvedic doctor V.A. Venugopal told us that preparing for pregnancy involves understanding that you are about to be of service to the world, to contribute something great through parenting a conscious child. Your "duty" involves adopting a healthy lifestyle in body and mind, and expanding your consciousness, because this self-development "affects the purity of the soul coming through." Closer to home, the indigenous Northern American traditions teach that this sacred aspect of parenting is the most important part of all, for all of creation has worked to bring the couple together at the behest of the child's spirit, who told the sacred beings it was her time to go to Earth. To honor this, a young person moving from adolescence into parenting years undergoes rites and initiations overseen by clan elders, which in various ways help the youth to release negativity, receive guidance, and honor life. For a woman, this involves understanding the power of her menstrual cycle and her connection to "Grandmother Moon" through lessons and rites led by the matriarchs. These help her to know the feminine as a profoundly generative force, centered around the creative reservoir of her womb.

Our exploration naturally brought us from the old ways to new ones, as we found guides and healers who may have been trained in traditional methods yet cognize knowledge about conception and motherhood in a wholly modern way. They opened our minds to often overlooked subjects, including the effect of trauma on a woman's readiness to conceive and the power that can come from healing it.

As we explored more of my own family's heritage, traditional Chinese medicine (TCM), we discovered layers of potential—and complexity! TCM sees the body as a complex network of organ systems and energy pathways, or meridians, that affect each other in myriad ways to subtly influence that sought-after state of fruit-bearing balance and harmony. To be frank, deciphering it is intimidating. Those who are expert in this medicine speak a language that is part literal and part super subtle; part about functions that are quantifiable and palpable, and part about the *energy* that drives those functions, something that is there but invisible, and thus harder to detect. TCM, like Ayurveda, takes years to learn and decades to master. Yet while it has layers of complexity, it is at its core a medicine that is alive in everyday life and rooted in a philosophy that sees health holistically; not only seeing our bodies, minds, and spirits as completely connected and mutually interdependent, but also as being in constant relationship with the greater rhythms and cycles of nature, and belonging to the universal field of life-giving energy.

And because of this holistic point of view, TCM's path of health and longevity offers universal insight about preparing for parenting that applies to every woman—and man—and that correlates with wisdom from other global traditions. In order to parse wisdom that could serve us on the path to mothering today, we pulled out the most important insights from TCM, put them into a blender with all the other global insights we'd discovered so far, and landed on three timeless directives for the preconception period.

I. conserve your fertility potential

You have a fertility potential that exists from the first whisper of your mothering potential, your first period, to your final ovulation and last period as you transition into menopause. Fertility potential exists naturally, yet it can be more awake at some times than others; because it is one expression of your total vitality and health, its brightness can get clouded or obscured depending on how hard you are pushing your body, what you are experiencing mentally and undergoing emotionally, and what level of care you've been giving yourself at every level, including the subtlest realms of your spirit. For all these reasons, it is something to start preserving, protecting, and nourishing as early as you are aware of it. When this becomes an ongoing lifestyle, you set the conditions for pregnancy to arise fairly straightforwardly. Furthermore, while fertility potential may lessen in potency as you get older, it doesn't disappear—the potential is there until menopause—but as you age, it likely requires extra support and care.

This notion of an always-present fertility potential that can be hidden or dimmed when your lifestyle gets off track and stress builds up, but that can also be uncovered and brought back into the light, is why in the traditional teachings, age isn't as limiting as mainstream understanding would lead us to believe and "infertility" seems to be a nonexistent term. Imbalances and temporary blocks that require patient and methodical treatment and lifestyle changes, yes; fixed or irreversible-sounding states of barrenness, no.

But where does this elusive-sounding "fertility potential" live, we wanted to know? In Chinese medicine, this potential is centered in the Kidney organ system, with two other organ systems, the Liver and Spleen, as crucial supporting players. Another two organ systems, the Lungs and Heart, are also involved. The Kidney, Liver, and Spleen are seen as the yin organ systems of the body; yin is the receptive aspect or principle of the creative energy that forms all matter, where yang is the active principle or aspect. Conception, as much as it is about actively growing a child, requires receiving—the sperm "catches the egg" and together they move into the "baby room," so the invitation must be there for new life to take residence within.

Organ systems in Chinese medicine are thought of a little differently from organs in the West; they refer not to just the physical organs, but a system of material and energetic function that influences both body and mind. On the one hand, your physical kidneys filter toxins from your body—an essential life-preserving function on its own; on the other, the Kidney system is said to house your willpower, to govern the balance of water and fire in your body, and to control your internal *chi* (the vital force or essential energy of aliveness) and the balance of yin and yang (the two paradoxical energies that comprise everything in nature). And, very importantly, your Kidneys house your jing. Jing doesn't translate easily into English. It's like a combination of your genetic potential and your lifestyle factors; it's described as an essence that governs how healthy you are, how well you age, and, not surprisingly, how fertile you are and how easily a woman conceives, carries a child, gives birth, and recovers. It's the treasure chest of your health that you inherit from your parents and then take care of throughout your life, spending it carefully, tending to the coffers through a balanced, positive lifestyle, good food, and cultivating joy and community, and that in return manifests as powerful reproductive potential. Most classical TCM practitioners say we cannot *add* to our jing, but we can take care of what we have so it remains strong; some vanguard healers see it differently—that we can add to it and compound it through superb diet, a full heart, and a joyous mind-set. Both agree that not spending it wildly through excesses in lifestyle or treating our bodies like unbreakable machines is paramount.

Imagine your jing or your ojas as a sacred jewel sitting inside a beautifully lit chamber. Your yin organs are its protectors, so you want to give them plenty of resources to do their jobs.

Because jing resides in the Kidneys, the terms are sometimes used interchangeably—a woman with strong jing will have strong Kidney chi and vice versa—and there is a correlation between jing and the Western understanding of adrenal energy, as the adrenal glands reside on top of the kidneys and produce bursts of energy under duress by secreting adrenaline and then cortisol. Like jing, adrenals can be easily maxed out by chronic stress, lack of sleep, dietary depletions or overindulgences, overuse of stimulants, and stresses from toxins, drugs, and other shocks to the system. They have only so much to give, and when we exhaust them and run them into the ground, our health can be hard to turn around. Just like with exhausted adrenals, it's said that when jing is depleted and weak, we age prematurely and get sick more often—our whole system is thrown out of whack.

But jing is more magical and wider-reaching than adrenal function; ancient texts describe this essence in similar ways to Ayurveda's ojas, the subtlest substance of life, which manifests as eggs and sperm and as such is the "reproductive essence" of women *and* men. Which is why—and this is important to highlight, because it is all too often overlooked—TCM experts say that when fertility issues arise, 40 to 50 percent of the time it's the male who needs help to rebalance and fortify. It's also deeply significant because jing is the treasure we inherit from our parents—the size of the inheritance is determined by their states of health *at the moment of conception.* Ergo, it's the treasure that *we* then pass on to our children, one that will have a massive impact on their vitality, resilience, and longevity. Thus, we want to tend to our jing (and the Kidney system that houses it) with respect and care, knowing our choices today impact our future offspring's well-being tomorrow.

This isn't as out-there as it may seem; it's an earlier expression of what today's science is now describing as epigenetics, the ways lifestyle factors influence how our genes express, and how the health and lifestyle of one generation influences the next generation's predisposition to disease (and even the generation's after that). The "Jing Thing," as I like to call it, is why the Kidney organ system is seen to be the foundation of life and why in TCM—and in grandmothers' kitchens—there is such an emphasis on nourishing and strengthening the Kidneys through food, and on becoming aware of when you feel depleted and worn out, because those sensations are your Kidneys telling you they're tired. As one of our wise ones, the Winnipeg-based master herbalist Chad Cornell, describes it, that fatigue is the message that your Duracell pack, your battery of jing, which you also pass on to your children, is running low. In a sense, living moderately today, dipping into the treasure chest wisely and not spending all the gold at once, is not only about safeguarding your own health, longevity, and yes, your beauty; it is your "service" to the child or children of your future. You are preserving your inheritance for them—the wealth of their health, so to speak!

To complete this micro-course in fertility potential, let's look just a little wider. The Liver organ system and its sister system, the Spleen, are also central to the rejuvenated and fortified state that supports a balanced menstrual cycle, smooth conception, and healthy pregnancy. The Spleen (which is commonly considered in tandem with the Stomach as one organ system; it corresponds with the Western understanding of the pancreas and to some practitioners, the master hypothalamus gland, too) works to make "strong blood" from the nutrients we ingest and to "hold" it in the blood vessels and create a healthy uterine lining; the Liver, as seen through TCM, helps to propel the blood around the body in healthy circulation, to "move" blood in a balanced way. As such, the Liver and Spleen help make the "baby room" warm, plush, and "well furnished" with a healthy uterine lining. They also play significant roles in establishing a healthy menstrual cycle. In traditional medicinal texts, the word "hormone" does not appear; it's a Western term coined at the start of the twentieth century. But the understanding of the cascades of signals and actions that happen within the body as a result of these biochemical messengers is similar. And we now understand how the physical function of the liver (and its sibling organ the gallbladder) includes digesting fats, the basic building blocks for hormones, from foods; it also breaks down old hormones, predominantly estrogen, that have served their purpose in one cycle, so that new hormones are made for the next, helping to maintain hormone balance. One of the very experienced TCM doctors in our maternal health circle, the fertility expert Danica Thornberry, describes the Liver and Spleen as lending "post-heaven support" to the Kidney-jing system—in other words, they let us add support to our "pre-heaven," or inherited, reserves via our own lifestyle choices in how we eat, live, and care for ourselves.

The ancient Daoists said that if a woman cycles in harmony with the moon, ovulating with the full moon and bleeding with the new moon, she is in tune with the universe and the cosmos. Traditionally speaking, a child conceived on the full moon will inherit greater jing, whereas a child conceived on the new moon will have less jing.

—LAUREN CURTAIN, women's health acupuncturist and Chinese medicine practitioner

The three yin organs that support our fertility potential all require care if we want to lay the groundwork for pregnancy. They can be easily taxed in modern existence, with its strongly yang nature. We can become depleted in Kidney energy or Kidney *chi* by working hard and handling demands without respite; our Liver *chi* can often become stagnant, not only from poor foods but from frustration, anger, and, as Danica says, the "constant comparison" women live under and, moreover, the stifled resentment this can breed. Meanwhile, the Spleen, an organ system that works best when we feel calm, soothed, and safe—the best conditions for digestion, as most of us know—can become overwhelmed by constant overthinking, obsessive worrying, or perfectionist tendencies.

Like three children with three distinct personalities, the Kidneys, Liver, and Spleen all need daily loving attention if they are to behave well! But here's the twist: there isn't one set way to do this. The traditions teach that we best stay in balance by observing subtle shifts and getting to know the signs that one area is needing support—even if at first this takes some guidance from others around ideal foods, routines, and behaviors. As our good friend the Vedic wellness expert Jillian Lavender shared with us, the old ways are not prescriptive; they're about knowing what's right for you in any given moment. "We don't say *no*," she shared. "In Ayurveda, we say *know*." It's about starting that conversation with your body early and, over time, getting to know it like a friend. *How's my Kidney energy doing—is it totally out of gas? How's my Liver—am I frustrated, quick to tip into irritation?* With practice, this curious listening is how we can start to maintain our balance and get to know our changing needs; eventually, it can lead us to become our own medicine woman.

2. fill your reserves

It used to be commonly understood that pregnancy takes a lot out of a woman's body; growing another life from her own blood and tissues requires an extraordinary amount of energy and raw materials. No wonder Danica Thornberry taught us the traditional precept that when chi (life-force energy) and blood (substance) are overflowing, and when there is an abundance of nourishment in the body, should sperm meet egg, conception will occur. But how many women really feel overflowing with energy and vitality, or brimming with too *much* high-grade nutrition? Today, it's becoming harder for busy women, constantly in a state of giving outward, to feel that way at the drop of a hat; it's harder still for second- and third-time mothers. We have to give our systems a prelude to pregnancy, a time to work up to it. For the healers we spoke with, there was a common wish: that no woman enter pregnancy in a depleted state. Conception might still occur, though not surprisingly it will be significantly harder if any of the trio of chronic stress, sleep deprivation, and nutritional deficiencies are present, for all these things disrupt the chemistry of reproduction. But as the author Catherine Shanahan, MD, describes in her book *Deep Nutrition*, if the maternal diet is lacking, particularly if a mom hasn't restored herself well after one pregnancy or if her diet is replete with damaging foods like sugars and vegetable oils, then the developing baby will take what it needs from the mother's body—even if that robs her bones of calcium or her brain of neurologically necessary fats, rendering her susceptible to bone deficiencies, memory or concentration issues, or postpartum depression. In the breastfeeding and maternal recovery phase that follows, her body's reserves will be tapped further still. But it needn't be this way; when the body is deeply nourished with whole foods in their natural state, with plenty of vitamins, minerals, and high-quality fats along with good protein sources, a woman builds up closer to that state of overflowing, brimming with strong blood and chi. In the simplest terms, the season *before* you become pregnant is the season to fill your reserves!

As someone who cooks for women before, during, and after pregnancy, I always turn to fresh, whole, colorful, unprocessed foods, in a natural and chemical-free state—you can almost feel how they are repositories of jing and ojas, charged with the energy of life. Because my artist's mind doesn't do well with scientific lists of nutrients, when building up reserves I serve the organs. As we'll see in Chapter 5, the Kidneys require fortifying foods—like sardines and shellfish, black beans, dark leafy greens, soaked walnuts, bone broth, bison, mineral-rich seaweed—and some healthy saturated fat from foods like lamb, high-quality eggs, and grass-fed butter to "pad the adrenals," as Danica likes to say. The Spleen thrives with foods like pumpkin, squash, yams, and grass-fed beef; the Liver loves lots of greens (especially bitter ones), cleansing beets, extra-virgin olive oil, and sour tastes, which soothe it. These foods are chock-full of the essential building materials that prepare parents-to-be and then give baby what he needs. When prepared in appropriate ways— often slow cooked to be easy to absorb, balanced in energetic temperatures (neither overly heating nor overly cooling to the body) and flavors, free of sugars, and not fried at high heat—they do their jobs brilliantly.

In the pre-pregnancy and recovery phase, good foods can be supported with herbs and plant-based tonics that help the body balance itself and often support hormones, too; herbs are even more helpful when prescribed by an

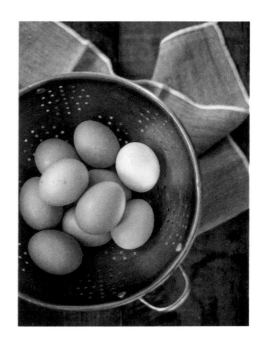

expert for your particular patterns of deficiency or excess. (During pregnancy and breastfeeding, it's better to stick to the classic pregnancy and lactation herbs and teas unless a trusted provider suggests otherwise.) This approach is less intellectual and intimidating, I've found, than trying to follow abstract lists of "must-eat" nutrients—omega-3s, magnesium, iodine—taped to the fridge. Everything about mothering adds complexity to your existence, so we want to keep this simple. I try always to remind women that filling the reserves starts with throwing out the bad stuff—clearing out the overly indulgent, fake, and factory-made foods first—and that in itself creates remarkable health benefits. When it comes to feeding myself and my mothers via my food delivery service, I live by another maxim of Auntie Ou's: "Too fancy food creates fancy trouble, needs fancy payment."

Moreover, the old ways teach us that *how* you eat is equally as important as *what* you eat. As the renowned subtle energy medicine practitioner Dr. Linda Lancaster tells my cowriter Amely—her patient and writing partner— on a frequent basis, it's not just what you eat; it's what your body *does* with what you eat. If your digestive system is weak or sluggish due to poorly chosen foods, high stress, and erratic eating habits—which Dr. Linda says is the case for most people today—you'll fail to get the potential nutrition out of your ingredients, even if they're top-notch! In other words, building up to a state of overflowing doesn't necessarily mean gorging on gallons of vitamin K–filled milk and cream or noshing on homemade jerky all day long, as some traditional dietary advice suggests. It means tending to the digestive system by giving the Liver and Spleen what they need to digest food well so that our bodies can capture the raw materials required, as we'll see in Chapter 3; it means eating seasonally, with building foods in winter complementing rejuvenating foods in spring; it means reducing some of the anxiety around eating "perfectly"—anxiety is a ruthless digestion-squelcher!—and knowing your body's tendencies, because what works well for one woman may not work quite so well for the next. At the MotherBees kitchen where we make our meals for moms, we view cooking holistically: tend to your roots by following traditions, enrich your soil with nutrient-filled fresh foods, and encourage blossoms and green leaves to flourish by bringing peace and gratitude to the table.

The goal is to embark on becoming deeply nourished, but without this causing more stress. With how much information is circulating today about eating, it's as easy to go overboard with nutrition as it is to overlook it. I've never forgotten the words of the Chinese medicine doctor and fertility expert Randine Lewis, in her book *The Infertility Cure*, that a woman's body must be *gently* nourished to bear fruit.

3. let yourself bloom

Over and again, as we talked to our wise ones, we were humbled by a simple teaching: allow yourself to feel the desire for a child strongly—really feel it!—take good care of yourself, and then, let it go. Auntie Ou voiced this as only she can: "As soon as you relax, baby room relaxes, soil is fertile, boom!" By contrast, however, she says, "Woman worry, no energy, hormone won't drop." You get the idea. Preparing for pregnancy isn't solely about putting a micro-focus on mom's ovaries and dad's sperm quality; that matters, but it's also about cultivating a broader state of well-being, and of gratitude and peace. We can help ourselves do that by putting attention on the health of our *whole life*, not only our reproductive organs; or, as Chad Cornell put it, not worrying just about getting enough folate, but asking, *Is my mind on board, is my heart on board?* Conceiving a child, growing a child, and growing into your own role as a mother involves the whole of you; preparation involves that, too. It's about creating the conditions for your flower to unfold fully, each and every petal turning outward to the sun.

So, as you "clear out" an energy-drink habit or paraben-filled body lotions, you might also consider clearing out habits of excessive worrying, overworking, or self-critiquing. As you "build up" reserves of fortifying food, you might also build up healthy relationships with friends and community—a necessary safety net for parenting, now more than ever—and even fortify your personal experience of unseen spiritual support, which could be through an inward-directed practice or simply a greater sense of trust that all will be well. You might even address layers of experiences around sex, partnership, and mothering that accumulate beneath the surface but tend to be invisible until you go digging, like grief, disappointment, sorrow, and trauma. The good news is that since everything in you is connected, when you physically clear out and build up your organ systems, your mental outlook, emotional energy, and even your sense of trust and faith can settle and return from any extremes, as the health of your organ systems directly affects how you think and feel. This doesn't make it suddenly easy to address the subtler blocks or sorrows that may be in there somewhere, but it will put you in a calmer and stronger place to face the shadows.

Fully blooming also involves a remembering of something so oft-stated it's almost a cliché: you are one facet of a cosmic whole. That doesn't mean you have to get all barefoot and groovy if it's not in your nature! Rather, remember what the old ways knew. Your body exists in a constantly shifting but harmonious relationship with the greater rhythms of light and dark and of sun and moon, with the cycles of the seasons and the shifts in weather. These rhythms and cycles all interact with your personal rhythms and cycles—the orchestration of hormones and even your energy production—and help you stay in balance. In Chapter 3, you'll be invited to lay down routines and rhythms in the everyday that help you work with, not against, larger patterns. Considering yourself a part of this grander scheme also opens the door to the great mystery of our powerful creative force, the beautiful brewing inside that can't fully be tracked with an ovulation app or known with full certainty.

So what do you get when you protect your fertility potential, fill your reserves, and let yourself bloom? We loved how the Australian doctor of Chinese medicine and women's wellness practitioner Lauren Curtain summed it up for us after we met her by following a trail of clues on Instagram—yes, we were scrolling, but we promise it wasn't late at night! "To tie all this together," she wrote, "for a woman to be ready to fall pregnant she will already have balance and joy in all areas of her health and life. Her body is balanced, she is nourished and eating regularly, she is getting deep restorative sleep at regular times, her digestion is harmonious, her skin is healthy, her mental state calm, she is at peace regardless of outcome, she has fulfilment and purpose in life already, her relationships are happy and joyful and she lives in a state of ease and flow." Wise words, indeed.

The world we live in is markedly different from the one the original medicine women knew. Now soils and the foods that grow in them are depleted of nutrition, and pollution is rampant, in forms they could barely have imagined. All sorts of factors are different, from the amount of time spent indoors to the amount of time spent awake to the number of toxins in so much of what we ingest, apply, and breathe. Yet the three universal directives still apply meaningfully, especially if we can view them through the lens of life as we know it today. Which is what we endeavored to do when we imagined five realms of exploration and discovery that a woman crosses on her passage of becoming a mother and that engage every part of her, not just the prudent part that might

As we weaved together the threads we gathered into the five realms of discovery, my cowriters and I received a message from the International Council of Thirteen Indigenous Grandmothers, a group that exists to share matriarchal knowledge from female elders around the globe. Their sentiment exquisitely captured the dance we found ourselves in, wanting to teach a solid foundation of self-care, yet wanting even more to help women do it with peace, trust, and calm. They wrote the following:

As you move through these changing times . . . be easy on yourself and be easy on one another. You are at the beginning of something new. You are learning a new way of being. You will find that you are working less in the yang modes that you are used to. You will stop working so hard at getting from point A to point B the way you have in the past, but instead, will spend more time experiencing yourself in the whole, and your place in it. Instead of traveling to a goal out there, you will voyage deeper into yourself. Your mother's grandmother knew how to do this. Your ancestors from long ago knew how to do this. They knew the power of the feminine principle . . . and because you carry their DNA in your body, this wisdom and this way of being is within you. Call on it. Call it up. Invite your ancestors in. As the yang-based habits and the decaying institutions on our planet begin to crumble, look up. A breeze is stirring. Feel the sun on your wings.

think to buy a bottle of prenatal vitamins. Awakening fertility is a process that marries the seen and the unseen, the practical and the mysterious, after all. Explore them at your own pace.

The first realm is Dreaming—there, you have an invitation to sink into a yielding, receptive state. The second is Preparing, where you begin to address the primary physical imbalances brought on by a modern lifestyle. The third is Clearing, where any blocks from the past are released and old hurts forgiven, and the power of your body's creative force is revealed. The fourth is Fortifying, which is where you fill your reserves by feeding yourself good food, and begin

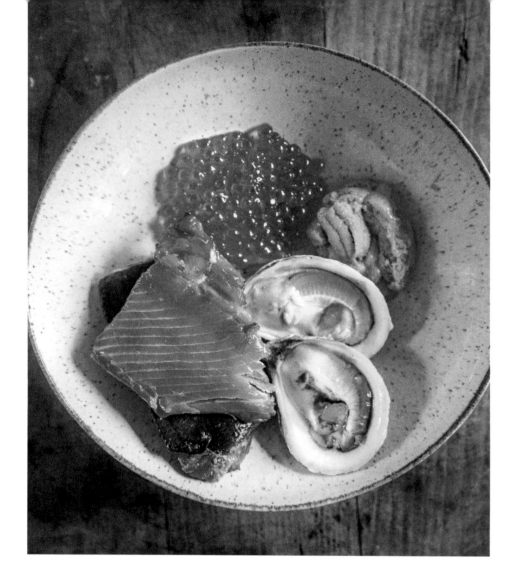

to tend to your body's needs for support by listening in with kindness. Finally, you arrive at Conceiving, where—you guessed it—you engage in the fun stuff in the hopes of "catching the egg," and find there's more to it than the mechanics, if you choose to experience it that way. We don't believe each woman *has* to engage in the realms that go beyond the physical—the basics of bodily health, Preparing and Fortifying—but they are there for you, even if only as a gesture or an invitation to think about something previously unconsidered.

Now to the big question. How long should this prematernal odyssey take? Since there's no set map, there's no rigid timeline, either. But when it comes to physically building up reserves of good nutrition, give yourself at the *minimum* three months (which is the approximate time it takes for sperm to generate and grow, and the approximate maturing time of each cycle's egg). Ideally, allot yourself six months, or better yet, gift yourself *years* of fortifying nourishment and balanced self-care! If you've stumbled onto this book many years before you hope to become a mother (or before you have even met a partner), congratulations, because it's never too early to tune in to your reproductive health and protect your fertility potential! If you're hoping to get started on your family, like, *yesterday*, see this book as an opportunity to check in. Is your garden already flourishing, popping with energy and ready for sowing your seeds? Or could a few months of tending to yourself now lead to a better growing season later?

By the way, these same questions apply as much to the male partner as the female, unless you are embarking on this voyage solo using a donor, a path we honor and respect. In traditional Chinese medicine, the man's fertility is evaluated with equal—and sometimes more—scrutiny than the female's. It's that important. If you're currently experiencing issues in your reproductive health that are getting you down, may what follows reassure you: *You are not broken.* There are myriad avenues to explore around the pressures that are put on our bodies, any one of which may help turn current imbalances around.

Taking this journey from Dreaming to Conceiving is not a fast track to pregnancy. Outcomes are never guaranteed, and besides, complete control is never an option. More than anything, awakening fertility is awakening the part of us that listens, responds to our body's needs, and trusts we have agency over our choices. Ultimately, that is how we enter the state of balance and harmony that takes us to the cusp of a new phase of life, inviting in the experiences of sharing a mother's love with others. The way that manifests—the *when, where, who,* and *how*—can often challenge us and surprise us equally, but they, too, are part of the waking up.

dreaming

When a woman arrives at Dr. Japa Khalsa's office in Española, New Mexico, seeking support for her conception journey, the physician and yogic therapist holds off on citing dos and don'ts or prescribing long lists of medicinal herbs. Instead, she invites the woman to stretch out on her treatment table. Acupuncture needles in hand, she bypasses traditional fertility points, heading first to a small area near the navel. This is the Palace of the Child, an energetic hotspot that represents the health of a woman's womb and serves as the source of the happiness that feeds her fertility. Looking up at the woman's smile for inspiration, she places two needles in a triangle formation around her navel to create another smile. For Japa, the road to motherhood starts here.

Though becoming pregnant can be influenced by many factors, a good handful of them physiological, Japa believes—as do many of our wise ones—that it is the woman's sense of contentment that most strongly influences all the others. When she places her needles at the Palace of the Child, she is connecting to the epicenter of the woman's happiness, honoring it as an essential aspect of her vitality and creative potential, and bringing attention to it if it has been lost or forgotten. When you are at peace with the life you're already living, your body and spirit are significantly more receptive and open, and you will be better prepared to navigate the potentially choppy waters of fertility, the rigors of pregnancy, and the demands of parenting.

The smile Japa forms with her needles also represents the woman's innocence and love. After all, it is likely her smile that attracted her partner to her, and, according to Japa, it is the smile, and the joy it expresses, that will bring her child to her through the ethers. By creating a grin on a woman's belly in the Palace of the Child, Japa honors the contentment that will serve as a sacred balm along a woman's potentially bumpy journey to motherhood. Activating this source of energy and happiness fortifies the woman for whatever lies ahead. Once a woman is zooming full-speed toward motherhood, her primal preparation devices will kick in, and she may be consumed with nesting, saving for college, and the rest of it. Starting off with a reserve of personal peace and happiness, even way before conception, will build a foundation that will hold a woman as she moves through each step of the process, regardless of the final destination.

As you lean into your own experience of becoming pregnant, you'll discover that bringing attention to your happiness is something that can easily get lost in a growing list of must-do items. As you turn your sights to eventual motherhood, there's lots to be done. All this conception stuff can be quite busy, indeed! You can be easily consumed by tracking fertility, doing research online, reading books, seeking outside support such as acupuncture, changing your diet, paying attention to your stress levels—and making love, of course. But keep in mind that there is an essential stillness at the heart of all this action. In TCM, one way of viewing pregnancy is as chi and blood that have become stuck, an essence of non-movement in the area of the womb. You are still living your life as an active, sentient being, but there is a grand reservoir of stillness growing inside you, a steadiness that represents who you really are at the essence of your being. As Japa tells her clients, the baby's spirit can sense the stillness of who you are, and conception occurs from that knowing place.

> The mother's job is to be receptive and open. She must be open to hear the calling of her child's soul.
>
> —JAPA KHALSA, doctor of Oriental medicine and certified yoga therapist

The stillness that is a future pregnancy can serve as the guiding light that reminds us that moving from one chapter of our lives to another—from our pre-pregnancy selves to pregnancy, motherhood, and beyond—is not something to be rushed into, an item to be crossed off a to-do list. Your mind may feel ready, but your body and spirit likely have some catching up to do. In nature, the seasons transition gradually from one to the next, and so we are designed to transition, too. Slowing down and lowering the volume on your life is the way to begin hearing what your physiology and emotions are trying to say, to attend to their needs, and to dream yourself into the future you long for. In an era of exaggerated doing, where most of us are rushing, thinking, watching, and scrolling ourselves away from who we really are, it requires conscious choice and a strong will to jump off the hamster wheel of action and just simmer down.

Can you resist checking your phone every five minutes? Choose to sit quietly instead of turning on the TV? Refuse to participate in the epidemic of busyness plaguing us all? At the end of the day, the only way to get to that quiet place is to actually get quiet.

At the heart of quiet is rest. Rest is a nonoptional part of the creation process, whether you're hoping to conceive or pursue another dream. You probably know that rest matters, if you read the wellness blogs and medical journals: we need rest, rest is good for us, rest is what it's all about. But you're not sure how to make it happen. If you're honest, real rest sounds like an impossible dream: eight hours of deep sleep a night, your worry-free head resting on a pillow of stardust, your ache-free body sinking into a mattress made of angels' wings. Like weekly massages and a live-in chef, this kind of sleep seems the stuff of fantasy, a luxury item reserved for Hollywood starlets and the royal family. But what if you looked at rest in a different way, through a different lens? Rather than giving up on actually achieving restorative sleep or relegating all rest to nighttime slumber, could you widen your lens to include other perspectives on restoration and rejuvenation? This doesn't mean you should avoid sleeping. You need restful sleep every night, and many hours of it. Lauren Curtain recommends going to bed between nine and ten every night, as the Kidney organ system, and the adrenal glands that live on them, are replenished and restored during the night. Staying up late can deplete Kidney essence over time.

You are a mother when you create anything.

—V.A. VENUGOPAL, Ayurvedic doctor

Women and rest go way back. The ancient traditions of Ayurveda and TCM understood that the masculine and feminine have different ways of replenishing our reserves and that we create in different ways, too. For women it is essential to decrease stress, action, and activity before we can attempt to create something new. We produce from a rested state. This can be a tough concept for many women to grasp, as modern society doesn't give us a lot of room to recharge. When we feel depleted we are encouraged to push through, to hurtle

Feeling droopy? Trade the caffeine or sugary pick-me-up for some quick shut-eye. Twenty-minute power naps can be your secret weapon, at home, at work, even in the car (while parked, obviously). Make a commitment to close your eyes and let go completely—rather than powering through a wall of fatigue. Set your alarm for twenty minutes and rest. If you don't fall asleep, you're still giving your body and mind a needed break.

ourselves into a second—or third, or fourth—wind. We may succeed, seeming to get it all done, but there is an energetic price that will always catch up with us. We'll look at rest as a form of physical stress release later in the book (rest is the antidote to stress, the archenemy of fertility), but here we invite you to see rest as a gateway to dreaming, a fundamental stepping stone along the path to pregnancy.

There's no way around it. To access your best self, produce your finest work, and maximize your creation potential—remember, making a baby is the greatest act of creation—you must make room for rest every day. It can seem like a handicap or a burden to be required to retreat and restore so regularly. It can feel risky and uncertain, indulgent even. If you don't work those extra hours, somebody else could get that promotion or raise; if you say no to those social plans, you may not be invited out again. But we see it as an opportunity. It is in this pulled-back, quiet state that your most significant dreaming takes place, and it's dreaming (and its cohort, imagining) that form the launch pad that will propel you toward the life you want.

You can dream only when you're still. Sure, your body can be moving through space as a passenger in a car or train, or propelling itself forward while strolling or practicing yoga, but your mind must be open and relaxed and your heart must be soft and receptive. Your truest longing, and the blocks that may be inhibiting it, can make themselves fully known only when you're calm and

DREAMING

undistracted. When you regularly put the brakes on *doing* (this includes all forms of thinking, worrying, planning, strategizing, and generally trying to figure things out), you start *being*. This will cultivate the mental and emotional spaciousness to allow you to sink into the deeper waters of who you are. It is here that you can touch into the felt sense (see page 56) of what you desire and begin to manifest it. Slowing down like this may take practice and some deft pivoting as you learn to shift your focus from the external, action-oriented tasks of pregnancy preparation—eating differently, moving more, and learning about your menstrual cycle—to the more inward-facing aspects of the process. Connecting with the quieter parts of yourself, the wordless realm of feelings, senses, and emotions, is equally important now.

Whether you're consumed with the desire to have a baby or just now exploring your feelings about motherhood—or if you're turning your sights to birthing a baby of another kind, like a personal or professional project—let this reflective, imaginative time before the next chapter begins be a period of conscious dreaming. Dreaming is a state you can inhabit fully. Rather than brush it aside as nothing more than a stopgap between here and there or a bridge to be raced over on your way from one way of being to another, we invite you to plant your feet here for a while.

In Dreaming, you're exploring the darker, more private, underground aspects of who you are, the parts of you that do not live on the surface, that you shield from the world. Clarissa Pinkola Estés, author of the bible of feminine introspection *Women Who Run with the Wolves*, calls this part of ourselves "the wild Self." She says: "When women reassert their relationship with the wildish nature, they are gifted with a

In the noise of modern life, we lose something: our ability to tap into our inner wisdom, which is a primary aspect of feminine consciousness. When we're able to de-excite and experience our essential nature, we're able to tune back into that wisdom and trust the subtle signals that nature is giving us.

—JILLIAN LAVENDER,
Vedic wellness expert

drift away

ACCESSING the open expansiveness of the relaxed mind can feel like an Olympian feat for those who spend most of their hours in the realm of thinking, processing, and problem-solving. But it is only with a relaxed mind, free to drift and meander, that you can daydream and imagine. There is an inherent state of simply being that begets this kind of dreaming—a definitive place of non-doing. To get there, you have to make some space in the jam-packed corridors of your brain; luckily, there are things you can do to support the process. Certain activities help to activate the brain state in which thinking simmers to a low hum, giving way to drifting and daydreaming. Walking is great for this, especially in nature. This is not a sweat-inducing trot, mind you, but a gentle stroll, where you notice the leaves crunching underfoot or the breeze caressing your face. As you move through the forest or down a quiet neighborhood street, thoughts will roll through your mind. Let them come. And let them go. If you notice a thought that feels good, carrying a positive energy that lifts you up or fills your heart, hold on to it for a few moments, and then let it go, too. More are right behind it. Freewriting or journaling with no goal or outcome is another way to access the beauty of the drifting mind. See the pen as an extension of your stream of consciousness; write without judgment or critique and resist editing what ends up on the page. (Need some inspiration? Try Morning Pages from *The Artist's Way* or 750words.com.) Another way to drift and dream is to lie flat on a bed or couch in the state between sleep and wakefulness. You can catch this wave just before opening your eyes upon waking in the morning, after a meditation session, or before you fall asleep at night.

If you have kids, claiming time to do nothing more than drift and dream can seem downright luxurious. As the primary caretakers for our tribe, it can feel selfish to do anything for ourselves, but counterintuitively, taking care of yourself makes you more available for others (in that inimitable "put your oxygen mask on first before helping others" way). Can you wake up before your crew rises to claim some time for yourself, or seek the support of others to check out of parenting duties for a bit? ⬡

permanent and internal watcher, a knower, a visionary, an oracle, an inspiratrice, an intuitive, a maker, a creator, an inventor, and a listener who guide, suggest, and urge vibrant life in the inner and outer worlds."

The wise ones say that before actively moving toward motherhood you should dedicate time to familiarizing yourself with your inner landscape and to dreaming about the things you long for—they see this nurturing of your inner self as a way to fortify the ecology that you will need to eventually sustain life. Let this phase of the preparation process be your season of yin. Where yang energy flows outward, the energy of action and outward motion, with bursts of heat and sparks of ambition, dreaming asks you to lean toward the yin. Yang is always present, ever in ebb and flow with yin, but now is the time to become cooler and quieter and look inward with softness and surrender. This unexplored part of yourself has a loamy richness, like a dense patch of forest that you slip into after sunbathing in an open field. This place is a retreat from the stimuli of the outside world, though it is teeming with life of its own: a quieter ecosystem of flora and fauna that can offer useful information about who you really are, if you have the courage to walk into it and if you're curious enough to peek under logs and dig into piles of fallen leaves.

In this dreaming phase, dedicate active time to imagining what you want while also getting real about the unaddressed mental, emotional, and spiritual blocks that may be slithering under those leaves and logs (more on that in Chapter 4, Clearing). We understand that when pregnancy is where you want to end up, those blocks may not be obvious even when you're staring directly at them. It can be challenging to proceed without a light to brighten the shadowy patches of your inner forest. An understanding about the nature of your belief system can help, acting as a torch to illuminate what's really going on in your mind and heart. Your beliefs are your entrenched understanding of how things are supposed to be. You may not realize that throughout the course of your lifetime you have developed a sturdy framework upon which your life unfolds. These are your beliefs. They are mostly unconscious and have a huge influence on what transpires in your world. Take pregnancy. It seems like a simple equation: pull the birth control, have sex when you're ovulating, and boom, you're pregnant. But sometimes it doesn't play out like that. Your desire to become a mother may be there, alive and kicking, setting off fireworks with its urgency, yet your beliefs are holding you back. Many women must cross a divide between the beliefs they established during the years when they didn't want to become pregnant and the beliefs that must be in place to move into motherhood. For some, it's less "mind the gap" and more like trekking across the Grand Canyon.

You likely spent decades dodging pregnancy. Like millions of modern women, becoming pregnant was the last thing you wanted to do, using every available method to make sure it didn't happen. You leaned on one or more forms of birth control, tracked your cycles for your least fertile days, and repeated an unconscious mantra on the daily: *I absolutely can't get pregnant.* Your thoughts are incredibly powerful. *I absolutely can't get pregnant.* When repeated over and over they become entrenched belief systems that can dictate the course of your life. *I absolutely can't get pregnant.* And when those thoughts are bolstered by the physiological barricade of birth control, you become an anti-pregnancy fortress. Now the tides have changed; you're a new person with new desires, ready to become a mother, but, dear one, beliefs are sturdy. It can take time to dismantle the walls that once kept you from motherhood.

Deep in the English countryside, another member of our circle of wise ones is considering new ways to scale those walls, pondering the effects of

> Most of us women have spent the majority of our reproductive lives telling our bodies not to become pregnant. Then one day, perhaps, we change our minds and our bodies have to follow suit. It might happen quickly and it might take some time. Trust in yourself, take care of yourself, and practice the art of surrender.
>
> —LACEY HAYNES, creator of School of Whole

the felt sense of motherhood

YOUR BRAIN may be thinking about having a baby nonstop, but are your body and heart on board? Try giving your imaginative juice to the felt sense of life as a new mom. Dreaming is about thinking, but it's also about feeling, and feeling is one of the most fundamental of manifestation techniques. It's simple and clear, and you don't have to be new age or spiritual to do it—and you don't need a lot of time. Throughout the day, simply imagine what it feels like to be a mother, but instead of doing so with thoughts alone, use your mind to transport you to the felt experience of being a mother. You could start with being pregnant, imagining your swollen belly, how it feels to pull your pants over your bump, how it feels to waddle down the street or to sink into a chair. Imagine what it feels like to hold your baby against your chest, her warmth against your skin, her peach-fuzz hair brushing against your chin. What does she smell like? How heavy is she in your arms? This is part visualization, part straight-up imagination. Use your mind to transport you to the place you long to be, but feel it in your body.

Dr. Venugopal wants you to expand on this feeling exercise and maximize the energy of pregnancy and birth by spending time with pregnant women and new mothers and their infants. Feel the fullness and love radiating from these women—you may feel the fatigue and depletion, too, also very real parts of motherhood—and find a place of joy and appreciation for their experiences. Dr. V. believes that once you deeply register what it feels like to be pregnant and a new mother, you will be preparing yourself to receive a similar experience by aligning your consciousness with that of a mother. It's the resonance factor, also seen in traditions that encourage a woman who hopes to become pregnant to eat foods that represent the female egg—orange segments, chicken eggs, and sesame seeds. Doing so primes your nervous system, entraining you to a future reality. ⬡

our beliefs on our desires, specifically as it relates to the woman's journey. Lacey Haynes is dedicated to empowering women to reclaim their sexuality, and their fertility, and she believes the path to pregnancy begins with rewriting the story that having a child will ruin your life. Since you were first sexually active you've been waging a war against sperm—blocking them with condoms and thwarting them with hormonal birth control pills. Lacey wants you to shift that inhospitable environment to something way more inviting by writing a new narrative about pregnancy and motherhood. You can be literal about it and put pen to paper to write out what your new desire looks like, using the present tense and its magical manifestation properties—*I have an easy conception and a glowing pregnancy. I am now holding my healthy baby against my chest*—and/or visual-

Should you feel "I'll only have joy if I get pregnant" or are despondent about what's *not* occurring yet, that is the Heart organ system speaking to you—in Chinese medicine, that's an empty Heart. The Heart is the anchor of the spirit, so we want to tend to it with foods that bring on joy—small doses of bitter coffee and bitter dark chocolate help, especially around your period, as bitter is the flavor associated with the Heart, as do green foods full of minerals. And we reframe things, asking, "What is bringing me joy and fulfillment already?"

—DANICA THORNBERRY,
doctor of acupuncture and Oriental medicine

ize yourself pregnant and mothering and start to translate these feelings into words, sharing your desire to be a mother with people in your life. These simple actions play a key role in turning the dial from "I must avoid pregnancy at all costs" to "I'm open and ready to conceive."

Active dreaming—that's anytime you daydream, imagine, fantasize, or visualize—is an essential aspect of your path toward pregnancy, because where attention goes, energy flows. Begin to notice where you put your attention.

Are you worrying about experiencing difficulty becoming pregnant? Are you scared about giving birth? Are you nervous about the sleepless nights that are an unavoidable part of new motherhood, about the time you'll need to take off from work, or about the changes that may happen to your relationship? Maybe you're decades ahead, already worrying about how you'll pay for college. When you are having worrisome, fearful, or anxious thoughts, you are giving your attention to worry, fear, and anxiety. When you are actively concerned about something, it may seem as if you are doing your due diligence to prevent that thing from happening. You're on it, vigilant and aware. But creation and manifestation don't operate like that. The longer you remain in those painful cycles, feeding anxious thoughts with more anxious thoughts, the more difficult it will be to break free. Hard thoughts cling to each other and multiply, expanding your fear exponentially, like a snowball rolling down a hill. Where a thought like *I don't have what it takes to get through childbirth* was once just a blip in your mind, when repeated over and over it becomes an established belief—and if not turned around, that belief drives new choices that support that belief, and before you know it, your beliefs really can become your reality.

> Living a life that you're not enjoying feels contracted and stagnant. If you want to plant the most epic creation in the center, but none of the other aspects have been attended to, it will be challenging. Make your life something that a seed would want to be planted in. Sometimes you need to shapeshift your life entirely to get out of a rut and not be so mired in the longing. It is from that place that dreaming can take place.
>
> —LACEY HAYNES

The exciting news is that you have control over your thoughts. You can decide to stop thinking negative thoughts and choose positive, empowering ones instead. It takes practice, but it's absolutely doable! Each time you hold your hand up to a negative thought, telling it that it's not welcome here, you create a new neural pathway in your brain, a new road for a positive thought to cruise down, instead of the well-worn road your negative thoughts have always traveled. Just as you'd strengthen a muscle with regular exercise, you must strengthen your capacity to choose better thoughts. You don't have to go from zero to sixty. If you feel as if you hold negative beliefs about pregnancy, childbirth, and motherhood, you don't have to try to change them right away. Start with something else instead, such as your beliefs about your finances (*I'm always broke* can transform into *I am rich in my health, my friends, and my family*) or your career (*I'm not good enough to get that promotion* can transform into *I deserve to get that promotion and will*). From there, you can move into more sensitive territory, like your future motherhood.

As you spend time feeling into what it's like to become pregnant and a mother, there's another side to explore as well—one that may be initially less enjoyable, but may lead to great rewards if you can stick with it. *Can you find the courage to ask yourself how you would feel if you never became a mother?* Pulling this question out of the dark corners can be terrifying, but the honest inquiry may lead you to the understanding that in clinging so fiercely to the desire for motherhood, you have vaporized from the life you have right now. Sometimes the number one thing standing between where you are now and your future as a mother is the desire for motherhood itself.

PARTNER DREAMS

Dreaming doesn't have to be a solo enterprise. Your partner will have a big role in your path toward, and through, motherhood. Don't leave him out. Take time to ask him about his hopes for parenthood—what he imagines it will look and feel like. Give him the space to express the secret desires that men aren't usually given room to share. If he doesn't have any, offer to help him dig a little deeper.

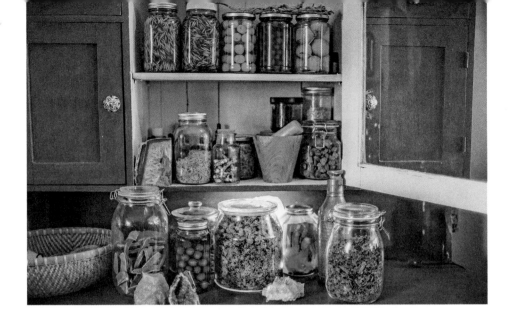

As you square off with this question, facing it directly, notice how tightly you are holding on to the dream of motherhood. (Please know that finding the courage to do so may take time. If you're struggling, don't do it alone. Seek help. Confide in a trusted friend or a therapist. Find the support you need to tackle this inquiry head on.) Does the idea of motherhood rest in a gentle embrace or is it more of a viselike grip? Dare yourself to be really honest with what you see there. Notice how you feel just sitting with the question. What happens in your body when you ask it? Is your heart heavy? Does your belly flip-flop? Is there tightness in your throat? Does your head throb or tingle? What you discover will help you see how much weight you have given to the idea of becoming a mother and will show you how you value yourself right now—without a child (or another child).

If upon reflection you find that you are gripping so fiercely to the dream of motherhood that it has eclipsed your ability to be peaceful and happy with what you have right now, it's a good idea to sit with that understanding. And then begin to explore the idea of creating a bit of space around the dream. When you release a little, you make space for nature to organize itself, without your desperately trying to control it. The spaciousness you generate in your mind and heart represents the softer, receptive, yin qualities that our experts attribute to conception. Don't worry! When you give some breathing room to your desire for motherhood, the dream won't escape; in fact, you're actually making more space for it to come in. Imagine cupping the dream of motherhood in your hand as if it's a baby bird you want to protect—with a light touch and gentle energy.

The way you relate to your desire to be a mother—again, do you have a white-knuckle hold on it?—can also show you if you are living what Lacey Haynes calls "a fertile life." For Lacey, and our other experts, fertility is about so much more than what's happening in your body or between your body and another's. It's about regarding your whole life as a landscape that you're inviting your baby into. A fertile life is a life appreciated. Not all the time, of course. You're not a princess in a Disney movie. But a good amount of the time. When you're living a fertile life, you regularly tap into the surge of energy that is born from inspiration. It's the way you feel when you talk about someone

In the Buddhist tradition, the word *sukha* is used to describe the deepest type of happiness that is independent of what is happening. It has to do with a kind of faith, a kind of trust that our heart can be with whatever comes our way. It gives us a confidence that is sometimes described as *the lion's roar*. It's the confidence that allows us to say, "No matter what life presents me, I can work with it." When that confidence is there, we take incredible joy in the moments of our lives. We are free to live life fully rather than resist and back off from a threat we perceive to be around the corner.

—"THE LION'S ROAR," TARA BRACH, PhD, spiritual teacher and author

you love, when you're in the flow of a creative project, or when you see a double rainbow arc across the sky after a rainstorm. This feeling can also be experienced when you touch into gratitude for the little things—the way a cup of soup warms your hands, a giggle shared with a friend, snuggling with your dog, sliding into crisp, clean sheets, or the way the sun hits the leaves in late afternoon. A fertile life is one ripe with appreciation for what you have right now—at

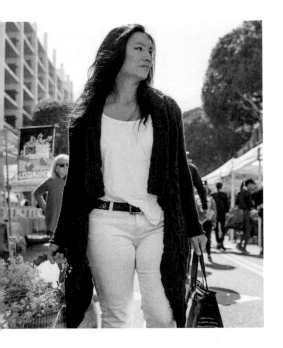

least most of the time. This may sound new age or too out-there, but it's actually a very pragmatic concept that will hold you up on your journey toward any new desire, motherhood or otherwise.

Japa Khalsa activates the Palace of the Child during her first acupuncture treatment with a new client because she understands that the first step toward fertility is to be happy *now*. By bringing attention to the energetic center of a woman's happiness, she sends an unspoken message: your own contentment will be your ally along the path to conception and will accompany you all the way through pregnancy, birth, and into motherhood. Easier said than done, for sure, especially when the heart longs for something other than what it has right now, but the motivation to get there is real. Happiness can take you where you want to go. Peace, joy, and contentment are receptive, open states of being, while worry, fear, and longing have constrictive qualities, cutting you off from the stream of goodness and abundance that is always there for you—which includes pregnancy and all the other things you want to happen in your life. When you widen the lens of your perspective to include your own happiness, you soften the fierce grip you have on the dream of motherhood, preventing it from being suffocated by your longing.

Enjoying yourself along the way is how you begin to build the foundation of your fertile life. This is why you continually hear stories of women who stopped "trying" to get pregnant, turning their attention to a new pet, a dream vacation, a creative pursuit, their relationship, even an adopted child, only to get pregnant soon after—a double win! It may seem counterintuitive, but by shifting their laser-beam focus from the dream of having a baby they made room for that baby to come in. When you tend to your own happiness, you make yourself

a more welcoming environment for creation. You can start by asking: *Is my contentment well watered and nourished?*

Many people connect happiness to an outside factor, living a life of "if onlys." *If only I had more money, I could be happy. If only I had a bigger house, I could be happy. If only I had a child, I could be happy.* But what if you could be happy right now? When you live a life of joy that is not predicated on any outside factor, you are truly free. You touch into true bliss and are living the most fertile life. This natural joy also feeds and protects your jing, your source of reproductive mojo. From there, anything is possible!

Cultivating a fertile life does not mean that you need to release the dream of motherhood. It's about finding balance. You can have a rich engagement with the life that you have right now while simultaneously nurturing a desire for something more. It's a "yes and" situation. *Yes,* I'm enjoying the life I'm living today *and* I look forward to what's waiting around the corner for me. You do not have to set your dreams down to be present with what you already have. This is the ultimate dance of adulthood: remaining content with where you are right now, while working toward your dreams. Can you have peace *and* motivation? Desire *and* contentment?

The dream is your guiding light: it illuminates the path that will undoubtedly have curves you can't see beyond and that will sometimes be bumpy and unfamiliar. You'll waver at times, losing your way and then coming back to center again. It's okay! Allow yourself to sink deeply into the unpredictable landscape of your wild nature. When you give your openhearted creator the permission to dream up the next chapter of your life, you will receive an invaluable gift in return: motivation to sustain you as you transform from one way of being to another.

Music, prayer, love, reading a good book, togetherness with those you love—all that makes you relaxed but energetic. Remember, in Ayurveda, we don't add energy; we only remove the blocks stopping the energy flow.

—V.A. VENUGOPAL

3

preparing

You've dreamed your way inward, into a realm where you've touched a receptive state of being and dropped into the quieter realms of feeling. Preparing has a more outward orientation—it's all about actions, nuts-and-bolts kind of stuff like assessing your present state of physical well-being and taking steps to shore up any weak spots (which we all have, by the way; it's called being a participant in modern life). Preparing involves rewinding to earlier in the physical part of the baby-making story and shifting the focus away from the offspring you hope to welcome one day, to tend to your own health and well-being, and that of your partner, first.

If you're the gardener hoping to produce a wonderful crop, think of Preparing as a necessary period of getting your field ready for the growing season ahead. As any good homesteader knows, you don't rush into planting, scattering seeds willy-nilly on whatever terrain happens to be there. You walk the land to evaluate its current condition, asking, How's the soil? Are there weeds galore that will hinder my own plants from growing? Are there rocks in the way that I need to remove? And you accept that a little manual labor invested in clearing away obstacles and, if necessary, remediating the soil—removing any impurities that may hinder healthy growth—goes a long way. The results may not seem staggering at first glance—*Wow, after all that work, all I see is a smooth and clear plot of empty land!*—but the wise gardener knows that under the surface the conditions are well set for building up and enriching the soil. There's a sequence. First, she prepares the field, then she builds it up with good nutrients (fortifying is the subject of Chapter 5, which focuses largely on food), and then—drumroll, please, or maybe a sexy soul-music soundtrack!—she is ready to sow. No surprise here, that's covered in Chapter 6, Conceiving.

There are so many ways to prepare your physical vessel for pregnancy. The subject of preconception health could involve endless investigations and programs of betterment at every level. But we're keeping it simple. What are the general aspects of physical well-being that, if you attend to them upfront, will create the best conditions for reproducing later? Which aspects help you preserve your jing (and protect your Kidney system's adrenal glands) and give those all-important organ systems, the Liver and the Spleen, the support they need to deliver vitality and health to your reproductive system? Obviously, every woman's body is different, as is every man's. But through talking with our wise ones, we landed on four key areas that are universally applicable and ask for our attention especially in our trying circumstances today, when the unrelenting pace of life can leave us quite disconnected from how our body is *really* doing down there, under our busy and filled-to-brimming heads.

In truth, all four areas are connected with each other, influencing and being influenced by the others. Nothing's separate, remember? Especially when talking about how stress, digestion, and reproduction interrelate. But separating them into quadrants helps give you four small health projects to work on— projects *you* can claim for yourself, even if friends aren't quite sure why they matter or wonder why you're turning down that second margarita.

The projects aren't necessarily about doing boot camps and dramatic health overhauls. Think of them more as getting into new routines that help you exist in a sweet spot between extremes—a sweet spot that is always slightly shifting, because our bodies are always in flux, never fixed, and one that is appropriate for your particular constitution or physical-mental makeup, matched to the way you tick. Chinese medicine doesn't start by giving one-size-fits-all doctrines. It seeks to address excess where excess shows up; to arrive at a place where your body's neither too heavy nor too thin, neither running too hot (which might mean inflamed) nor too cold (which you could experience as low thyroid levels). More specifically, it speaks of healthy organ systems being neither deficient nor in excess, and of the movement of energy and fluids being neither stagnant nor overactive. Addressing excesses also includes examining your lifestyle: the goal is to engage in a level of work and activity that is energetic and meaningful, but not exhausting; to eat a diet that is neither too heavy and clogging nor too light and airy; to move consciously and regularly but not dramatically overexercise; and to have an approach to life that is motivated but not manic (i.e., productive yang is balanced nicely with restorative yin). When you address all these things and more, you can help your body find its own sweet spot of balance and harmony—the state from which successful fruit-bearing can occur.

Of course, we're surrounded by excesses that simply didn't exist in earlier times. Overexposure to pollutants and poor foods, to stimulants like caffeine and alcohol, as well as chronic mental stressors, tobacco, pharmaceutical drugs (including hormonal birth control), and freewheeling cannabis use was not a pressing issue thousands of years ago. But the overall idea of tempering excess remains the same. Your body responds to every stimulus it encounters and interacts with, the helpful ones—like nutrients that build tissues or hormones, and sunlight that creates fertility-boosting vitamin D—and the challenging ones, too, from sedentary habits to man-made chemicals and nonnative radiation and more. If the challenge is greater than the body can deal with, a subtle imbalance can grow in one area of the body, which eventually ripples throughout, affecting other areas and beginning to manifest as "disharmony," as TCM calls it. Disharmony is a disturbance that, if not checked and corrected, can be the prelude to dysfunction of organ systems and energy networks and, eventually, physical illness. Obviously, we don't want to experience it if we can avoid it.

These overexposures matter enormously today because hormones—the natural chemical messengers that coordinate every activity in your body, including, and most sophisticatedly in our opinion, reproduction—are extraordinarily sensitive. So are the eggs in your ovaries—which, once damaged, are not replaced—and your partner's sperm, which alas doesn't get nearly enough attention given how easily lifestyle and environmental factors can negatively affect it (even innocuous-seeming factors, like a few relaxing cocktails and a hot bath). It would be naïve to pretend that we're not living in unnatural times in which both women's and men's fertility potential is under extra pressure. All the more reason to get clear on all the interferences we interact with daily and reduce them wherever possible, putting a little elbow grease into "pulling the weeds and clearing the rocks" from your physical field. (This is especially true if you or your partner is on the older side—experts disagree on what "older" means, but for the sake of consensus let's say mid-thirties onward—because egg and sperm quality do weaken, so give them all the help they can get!) Then, if you have tipped away from the sweet spot or even fallen into extremes, you can harness your body's miraculous ability to find its way back into balance. Sometimes when you don't feel well or you discover some part of your whole system has gotten off track, it can feel scary. But know that your physical design comes with an incredible knack: to come back into homeostasis—internally derived stability—if obstacles to good functioning are removed and the right things are given, in more or less the right amounts.

The way into this state of stability, teach the traditional health models, is routine. Consistent daily routines around eating and sleeping, movement and rest, efforting outward and diving inward, as well as seasonal routines of eating denser foods versus clarifying ones, all act to support a solid state of health, just as strong foundational pillars hold up a structure. (Which is particularly helpful in this "vata"-dominated age; vata, according to Ayurveda, is the air element, responsible for movement. Existing amid nonstop information, hyperconnectivity, and frenetic activity can make us especially ungrounded.) Routines, as Kerala's Dr. Venugopal made sure to reiterate when we asked him, help you embody the ineffable but all-important health-giving quality he calls "smoothness" (which itself is such a beautifully nonclinical word, describing a way of being more than a data set of perfect blood-test results). Smooth, consistent routines ground you so that you can relax into your healthy lifestyle— tweaking or adjusting it, or letting loose here and there—rather than clinging to a diet, exercise, or self-care regimen rigidly or fearfully, unable to adapt. Dr. V also emphasized that mastering "smooth habits" before you become a mother is just plain common sense. Lay down good, sturdy routines for managing stress, eating in ways your body digests well, and committing to sleeping soundly and long enough for your adrenals to restore—or to preserve your jing, depending on which way you see it—and you construct a robust and inner-derived stability

Smoothness comes from living in sync with natural rhythms (like light and dark cycles) rather than fighting against them; spending time in nature and in gratitude; tending to digestion and devoting moments to pure quiet, both of which together create the physiological equilibrium that ripples upward from the belly to a balanced mind-set, helping you find ease and joy in daily life more often than friction.

GET YOUR SPENDING IN ORDER

Unless you've been refining and recalibrating your lifestyle for some time, Preparing almost certainly involves getting your spending habits in order so that you're in a stable place to start a family. We're not talking financial spending in this instance, but getting a handle on the physiological overspending that occurs when you borrow more energy from your treasure chest of jing than your inheritance allows. Living to excess, be it by consuming too many poor-quality foods (or foods your body doesn't tolerate), pushing yourself to meet demands without resting (hello, gritted teeth and adrenaline!), or too much partying and too many late nights, forces you to withdraw energetic funds from your jing account in order to adapt to all the stressors. This might not seem to make much of a dent when you're young, but over time the withdrawals add up and an unbalanced lifestyle can deplete the trust fund that your parents gave to you—and hoped you'd save to pass on and that would also support you as you age. However, a balanced lifestyle based on routines and healthy habits helps to keep your reserve of jing brimming full and available to fund energy-intensive activities like healing, regeneration, and reproduction.

The lifestyle changes you make when you Prepare help you actively curtail any overspending so you don't enter into your childbearing years with low reserves or, worse, in debt and hustling to pay off your creditors at the same time as you're trying to create a new enterprise—a family! That's a situation you want to avoid, because if you start off depleted, the demands of mothering can cause your energy systems, your immunity, and consequently your outlook and mood to crash. Then, already tired and giving your all to your new family, it can be quite a bit harder to turn the situation around. The motto of Preparing? Don't cheat your body of what it needs to thrive; pay off your debts first!

that will support you on the unpredictable (and undeniably demanding) ride that follows.

And if you take a more left-brain perspective, don't worry. Smoothness and routine as we understand them do correlate with better health markers, things you can actually measure and discuss with your Western-trained care provider, like balanced cortisol levels, blood sugar, and thyroid markers.

Preparing your field for pregnancy is not significantly different from adopting a healthy lifestyle in general; it's just got a few distinct tweaks related to the unique circumstances around reproduction. If you've been postponing tying up any loose ends in your health or committing to lifestyle improvements, let the dream that you just envisioned motivate you now. There's no better reason to get to know your body well and establish reliable, supportive routines than the desire for a healthy baby! You might find that a light investigation into one area of Preparing is all that's required to find your equilibrium, while a deeper dive may be warranted in another. Rest assured that if you're familiar with, and doing basic maintenance in, all four areas before you hope to conceive, you'll be ahead of the game. Furthermore, bringing your partner in on the project will pay off double, not only because it's been shown to be far easier to optimize health when doing it with someone else, but also because it ensures that he also cleans up his act. To do the obvious math, sperm contributes 50 percent of the DNA to this project, and the quality of that DNA affects every step of the process (including how successfully a fertilized egg becomes a viable, lasting pregnancy). Preparing the man's field is equally important.

In Chapter 5, you'll read a lot more about food, which is often seen as the place to begin when you want to instill better health. Food matters—a lot—but in Preparing, you start somewhere subtler than that, by learning to speak the language of your menstrual cycle. It's remarkably simple, can start as soon as you think to do it, and requires no investment or accoutrements. And it is the way in to a deep and empowered connection with your body and your reproductive center that has the potential to hold you through the entire arc of what wisdom keepers call the three feminine initiations: Maiden, Mother, Crone.

In a sunny office just south of Melbourne, Australia, Lauren Curtain teaches her clients to interpret the messages from their bodies by tracking changes in their temperature, their cervical mucus, and their cervical position. This practitioner of TCM specializes in women's health, and to her, the surge of interest in learning all things menstrual is ridiculously exciting. She's part of a new wave of practitioners and educators helping women of all ages remember what has been largely forgotten: that they can have agency over their health, and even—over time—become their own medicine women, by paying close attention to when and how they ovulate and menstruate, and to the signs and symptoms that come with both.

If you visit a practitioner like Lauren, whether for help with fertility or for a general women's health evaluation, questions about your menstrual cycle will be the first thing you get. Do you know how long your cycle is each month—from the first day of one period until the day before the next? Do you know when you are ovulating? How many days do you bleed, and do you have any discomfort around that time, and does that change from month to month? What is your blood flow like, and its color? All these things can give clues to how your different organ systems are doing or indicate deficiencies or excesses that could lead to dysfunction. Small-seeming details they may be, but to Lauren, they're signposts pointing to areas where your diet and lifestyle may be out of balance and require some extra care. Many clots in your menstrual blood can indicate Liver chi stagnation and a buildup of heat from processed foods, pollution, or frustration; scant bleeding can indicate Kidney chi deficiency and possible fatigue, malnourishment, and poor sleep. Erratic spotting before your period can be a red flag, so to speak, that the Spleen is weak, anemic even, and not "holding on to" blood. It's saying, "Give me some gentle foods and warmth and make me feel safe!" And if you listen, the Spleen will help furnish your baby room (your uterus or womb) with a plush, inviting lining.

These things matter whether you want to ever have a baby or not. You need to be nourished and energized, to efficiently clear waste and toxins, and to be able to absorb food to live a long, healthy life! You need your major sex hormones, estrogen and progesterone, to be optimized and in balance in order to support many aspects of your health, from bone density, resistance to cancer, and resilience against today's "diseases of civilization" (diabetes, cardiovascular disease, high blood pressure), to your mental function and everyday mood. But these clues and indicators come into special focus if conception is on the horizon. At the most obvious level, tracking your menstrual cycle empowers you to know exactly when your fertile window is—a series of around five days leading up to the fairly brief yet awe-inspiring phenomenon that is ovulation. Ovulation is not always as mathematical an event as our linear minds want it to be—it doesn't always happen on day fourteen of the cycle on the dot. It's also susceptible to being delayed, or even disappearing temporarily, should your lifestyle fall into extremes. So you want the tools to track it, or else when it's go time, no matter how much you've got the other ducks in a row (like good nutrition and low stress), you will be shooting in the dark (so to speak). This takes on extra significance as you get older, as the fertile window can shrink. Learning the cycle lexicon and your body's own unique expression of it (because every body is slightly different) will also

> Women are cyclical, not linear.
>
> —LAUREN CURTAIN

empower you to safely shift off hormonal birth control, if you're using it, well ahead of the moment when you want to actively invite sperm to meet egg. And, should you face challenges later on your fertility journey, you will be well versed in what might be happening down there, armed with valuable data you've gathered by tracking your cycles. This can help you feel confident as you investigate any imbalances, either alone or with a trusted practitioner or team.

And don't forget the subtler but equally empowering reason to turn toward your reproductive system's rhythms. You can shift your mind-set a full 180 and rewrite your relationship with your period and even, maybe, your womanhood. For a lot of us, our cycle gets our attention for a scarce few days each month when we bleed—and even then, we might barely interact with it. The standard-issue response? Tampons inserted quickly to carry the blood away,

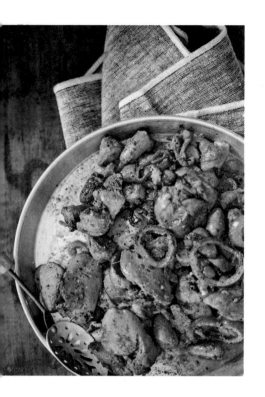

a painkiller popped if required, and a vague sense of inconvenience or perhaps even dread. But other than that, we try our mightiest not to let our body's releasing interrupt regular programming; through the force of our minds, we override the body and make life proceed as normal. (Of course, for many women, discomfort and bleeding can be significantly greater than this.) For the rest of the month, our menstrual cycle might be clicking away in the far background, out of sight, out of mind, unless we're actively using a tracking-based contraceptive method such as Fertility Awareness Method (FAM). And even then, what's actually going on between period and ovulation can be a bit of a mystery.

It needn't be that way. A cursory understanding of the phases of menstruation and what each needs to function smoothly—there's that word again—can be the start of a whole new chapter of self-knowing, because it can help you connect the dots between your lifestyle and your fertility, helping "make the case" for adopting balanced self-care routines. It can help to illuminate how your responses to stress, the condition of your digestive system, and the quality of the food you eat can make conception, pregnancy, and recovery a smoother journey or a rougher ride. And subtly, but so beautifully, it can help you embrace what Lauren loves to point out: as a woman, you are cyclical, not linear! Sure, all of society asks you to push forward in the same manner, at the same pace, impervious to fluctuations—in true linear style—but as a woman, your nature is different. Every part of your biology has set you up to move through life a little more circuitously, feeling ebbs and flows in your energy, shifts in your mental state, and changes in your emotions. Your very nature is to peak and relax, to open and close, to proliferate and release.

phases of the cycle

The more you learn about your cycle, the more empowered you feel. Maybe you remember the rush you felt when you first discovered you can't get pregnant every day of the month—who knew! But there's a lot more to learn than that. Did you know that in the underdiscussed world of menstruation, what we think of as indisputable truths are often quasi-myths? Like that cycles "should" be twenty-eight days or that periods are uncomfortable and painful, just because. It's a complex subject, but here's a CliffsNotes version of the key points.

The cycle starts on the first day of your period—you count that as day one—and thus starts the first of your cycle's two phases, the follicular phase. This is the *pre*ovulation phase, and at the start of it, your uterus sheds its lining because there is no fertilized egg implanted. Nobody's moving into the baby room this month, and the lining can be cleared and released as flowing blood, for it will renew again soon. About 70 percent of the lining typically is shed in the first day or two of bleeding, and then it slowly tapers off. If you have a Chinese auntie in your family, they'll cluck at you to drink hot water or green tea in the days before and during this event so the warmth and hydration can help the blood release smoothly, and they'll shoot you a death glare if you consume icy foods or drinks or sugar, all of which, they say, hinder the flow and cause cramping.

Your period is an example of the body's "slow yin" state as blood is moving for release—blood (substance) and movement (quality) are two expressions of yin. As such, when this shedding occurs, extra rest and quiet time is warranted—even if it's only an evening or two of quiet time, or pressing pause on afterwork activities (see "A Red Tent Day" on page 160)—though truthfully your body would delight if you actually got a few days to yourself, unplugged and, ideally, in nature. (Some warm soup with iron-rich ingredients would go down nicely, too.) In Ayurveda, menstruation is described as one of the major times that the downward-moving energy in the body, known as *apana vata*, is predominant. (Daily elimination, aka pooping, and giving birth are others.) Staying super engaged in busyness or allowing stress to take over your mind can cause its balancing counterpart, the upward-moving energy called *prana vata*, to resource energy from down below—stealing it, in a sense, and robbing menstruation of the energy it needs to happen easefully. Ayurveda was onto this millennia before our modern understanding of stress and physiology: like TCM, it teaches how slowing down a little during menstruation will help your whole system work in harmony. Part of this heightened connection to yourself may mean letting yourself *experience* your flow physically by switching from a tampon to a pad or period panties. How many of us spend years using tampons and never actually feel the sensation of blood releasing or see the variation in color and flow?

The rest of the follicular phase is all about building up to your reproductive system's great hurrah: ovulation. Two of the glands that coordinate hormone messaging, your hypothalamus and pituitary, signal the ovaries to "ripen" a clutch of eggs in small sacs called follicles. (To get technical, this happens via follicle stimulating hormone [FSH] and luteal hormone [LH].) Your follicles start the flow of estrogen hormone, thickening the inner layer of the uterus lining and rebuilding it once your period is complete. Now everything starts to really ramp up! About a week to ten days after your period ends, you feel some moistness around your vulva. That's because the glands in your cervix—the narrow neck of the uterus that sits in the vagina and can open and close—have received the message to make cervical mucus, a wonder substance that helps sperm in their quest to meet an egg. Your fertile window is opening!

Let's talk about mucus for a minute. For an older generation who were taught their lady parts were unmentionable, vulvas and mucus might be an uncomfortably

When we attune to the rhythm of Grandmother Moon, we step into remembrance of our divine feminine blueprint, recognize our place in the natural world, feel connected with women everywhere, and embody our truth from the sacred source of love.

—ACHINTYA DEVI,
founder of Goddess Rising Mystery School and Global Sisterhood

If connecting to apana vata or "downward energy" sounds heady (or hard), practice it physically. Neesha Zollinger, an Anusara yoga instructor in Jackson, Wyoming, recommends doing deep squats—aka yogic squats, or malasana—to enliven the oft-forgotten apana vata, allowing it the same importance as ever-thinking prana vata. "A deep squat is the most supportive way to get downward energy flowing," she says. "You want to move the bones to a place where energy, and breath, can go down as much as it goes up." Unlike other yoga poses requiring precision and agility, squats adapt to the person doing them. Your body will naturally assume the squat that is right for you, and regardless of how it looks, the pose will benefit you greatly. Squatting helps to correct the alignment in your hips and thighs, massages your organs, and opens up the pelvic floor, descending it as much as 30 percent—useful for those of us (most of us) who tend to be pulled up and tight. If you're not a regular squatter, the position can feel quite intense. You can turn the volume down on the sensation by placing a yoga brick under your butt for added support and leaning your back against a wall. It also helps to turn your feet out. If possible, sink into the pose several times a day while you focus on taking deep, downward breaths.

sticky subject (we had to go there). Thankfully today we're accelerating past patriarchal shame. Cervical mucus is glorious! This juicy message tells you pretty clearly when you learn to identify it and often quite abundantly, *You're fertile!* Cervical mucus helps sperm survive long enough inside you to get their shot at meeting their other half (your egg). It hosts them comfortably, if you will, while they're waiting for the diva to show up. It's because of mucus that your "fertile window" is longer than the short period that an egg spends outside of the ovary before dissolving, about six days on average. (The math: sperm tend to live up to five days; then add in another day for the time your egg hangs out after ovulation.) How does it do this? First, your vagina's pH is too acidic for sperm; mucus has an alkaline pH that suits sperm perfectly. Second, its structure has channels that help sperm swim upward toward the temporarily open, yielding cervix and through to the fallopian tubes. Third, its chemical nature even alters the sperm head so it can penetrate an egg.

One more detail about mucus. You'll notice the first few days you see and feel mucus, it's creamy and white, almost like lotion. But then it changes slightly, becoming clear, almost like a thin version of egg white. Hold it between your fingers and experience its texture: you'll find it stretches rather than feeling sticky or tacky. This is your *peak* mucus, secreted as your estrogen peaks, and it's extra supportive to sperm. Peak mucus is your signal that estrogen levels are high and ovulation is approaching. Though you can't see it, your rising estrogen has also caused your cervix to change position in anticipation, opening and

READING THE SIGNS

The East-West fertility physicians of New York City's Yinova Center share how the color and flow of your menstrual blood can give you clues to your state of balance:

Crimson, like red wine or pomegranate juice, with a fluid flow	Balanced hormones
Pale and watery	Spleen deficiency
Dark and clotted	Liver chi stagnation and blood stasis
Superbright red, mucus-thick	Excess heat, inflammation (seek medical help if any pain, fever, or discharge, in case of infection)
Deep purple, large clots	Blood stasis (if persistent may indicate endometriosis or fibroids)

softening and sitting higher in your vagina—the gate has opened for the sperm. (You can feel this with a clean ring finger inserted gently.) About a day and a half before ovulation, your pituitary gland sends a message to one follicle: *Get ready to release your egg!* (Ovulation predictor kits measure this surge in luteal hormone.) Your body cools very slightly. Chances are you are around day twelve or fourteen of your cycle. It's a good time to check any super-sedentary slump you may be in. You want to optimize circulation, not constrain it—get moving!

Why is this so exciting? Not just because a testosterone surge is likely making you horny. And not only because ovulation is a master event in your body that allows critical health-giving hormones to exist (hurray!). But also because this surging and opening is a rush of yang energy indicating that the cycle is about to make a big shift. Your body is raising its volume and saying, *If you're ready to make a mini me, the creative forces are building, so get on it!* Time is of the essence, because once the egg (or occasionally, two fraternal-twin-making eggs) bursts from its follicle, its presence is fleeting. It will hang out for a maximum of one twenty-four-hour cycle (and sometimes just twelve hours) before dissolving if not fertilized.

You've now shifted from the yin half of your cycle to the yang half, the luteal or post-ovulation phase. Hopefully you've been eating well, because all this activity requires energy. But it also gives you energy. Ovulation is a time of peaking, a time to, as Lauren Curtain puts it, feel great and "Get sh*t done!" And if your system is in balance, the feel-good effect can carry through the luteal phase, partly because the now-empty follicle on the ovary (called the corpus luteum, hence the name of this phase) produces progesterone. Like mucus, progesterone should be given a parade and high fives. This magical female sex hormone helps you hold a pregnancy and also counters anxiety, keeps your spirits up, helps prevent bloating and water retention, and, when there's enough of it, balances estrogen in your system so you don't get PMS. In this post-ovulation surge, progesterone dries up the cervical fluid and closes the cervix—the sign in the fertile window now says CLOSED—and warms your body temperature—so that the baby room is nice and warm—which will now stay raised for the rest of the cycle. (Hence, seeing your body temperature shift can help you confirm if and when ovulation has taken place.) Progesterone also works hard behind the scenes making your uterine lining super welcoming for an incoming blastocyst (the fertilized egg that will soon become an embryo). It takes this blastocyst about a week to travel to the uterus, and during that time progesterone is enriching the lining nicely, making it spongy and helping it secrete fluids the developing embryo will need. Moving into the baby room, aka implanting into the uterine lining, takes around another week. If an egg has not been fertilized or successfully implanted, the ovaries' secretion of estrogen and progesterone ceases and the uterine lining is cast off, starting a new cycle. Whew! The whole cycle *likely* took around twenty-nine days, though a give or take of five to six days shorter or longer is actually considered relatively normal. If this is your consistent pattern, you are otherwise symptom free, and you can confirm ovulation is occurring. (Advanced note: As you track your cycle length, pay attention to the length of your luteal phase. When preparing a woman for pregnancy, Lauren helps women achieve a fourteen-day luteal phase, indicating healthy hormone balance and stronger chances of success in conceiving and holding the pregnancy. When the luteal phase is eleven days or shorter, issues are more likely to arise.)

Why go into so much detail here, you ask? For one thing, the lifestyle you lead preconception directly impacts the way your body can keep estrogen and progesterone in balance, so that this coordination of events can occur relatively smoothly. Hormones are made from the food you eat, after all—cholesterol is the main building block!—and as you'll read below, you can help your body clear old hormones to maintain balance, or inadvertently hinder it, depending on how well you support liver function and elimination. The amount of pollutants you face daily, the levels of stress and amount of sleep, and even the darkness in your bedroom can all affect this intricate dance.

Understanding and tracking your cycle helps you see patterns of repeating imbalance and identify areas of weakness that can affect your fertility significantly. Lauren says that egg quality and follicular development, as well as luteal phase length, is highly influenced by the diet, lifestyle, medications, and self-care practices (like acupuncture) we follow during the three months leading

leading up to each ovulation. This is why three months of rebalancing and targeted care can help mild imbalances to correct and irregularities in ovulation or cycle phase length to regulate. When disharmonies have been building up for a while, however, correcting will likely take extra time. It's beyond the scope of this chapter to describe all possible imbalances; we recommend that all women who are menstruating, of all ages and life stages, lean on a terrific resource, *The Fifth Vital Sign* by Lisa Hendrickson-Jack. She not only goes into greater depth about the cycle but explains the root causes of common imbalances, including low thyroid levels, polycystic ovary syndrome (PCOS), endometriosis, hypothalamic amenorrhea, digestive and bowel issues such as SIBO and IBS, and underlying infections such as Lyme disease or Epstein-Barr virus. All of these can be addressed through steady care, usually with a supportive practitioner who uses a whole-systems approach—be that TCM or functional medicine with a special knowledge of endocrinology—so that your *whole* health, and ergo your menstrual-cycle health, can find its way back to balance.

MASTERING YOUR FERTILITY

The three signs—cervical mucus, waking temperature (aka BBT or basal body temperature), and cervix position—are the basis of the Fertility Awareness Method, a time-tested, natural system for tracking when you are fertile and when you're not. When used carefully, and ideally learned from a trained practitioner, it has a very high accuracy rate of both prediction and prevention, and lets your body cycle naturally—no potentially disruptive synthetic hormones involved. If it resonates as right for you, give yourself a few months to really get in the swing of it, using barrier methods of contraception as backup. While many books and websites now teach FAM, consider taking an in-person class, please! A host of apps and trackers such as Natural Cycles, Glow, Daysy, and Kindara now exist to let you do your tracking digitally.

POST PILL

Hormonal contraceptives such as the pill, the patch, and injectables have revolutionized society in so many ways. But with a cost. They also change your cycle. Most hormonal contraceptives use synthetic versions of estrogen and progesterone to prevent your ovaries from releasing eggs—TCM says the eggs have "gone quiet"—to thicken mucus so sperm can't swim to its destination, and to thin your uterine lining to prevent implantation. The "bleeding" you experience on the pill is not a true menstrual period, magically occurring on a naturally regulated twenty-eight-day cycle; it's a withdrawal bleed caused by taking sugar pills for five days. By suddenly taking away the hormones, your body hears, "Shed the thin lining," but the natural signaling between the hypothalamus, pituitary, and ovaries (the HPO axis) is disrupted. So it's probably not surprising that when you go off the pill hoping to conceive, hormone signaling can take a while to realign. This is especially true if you've been on the pill or another hormonal birth control to reduce symptoms around your period; chances are that any underlying imbalances are still there—and likely have been exacerbated. One of our favorite wise women, the medical doctor, midwife, and herbalist Aviva Romm has written that statistically, most women regain hormonal balance within three months of coming off the pill. But for others, regulating can take considerably longer—up to a year or more. Nutritional depletion, increased inflammation, microbiome changes, impaired gut health, compromised thyroid and liver function, and more tend to affect every woman in this situation to varying degrees, so the more time you can give yourself to prepare and fortify, the better. The book *Beyond the Pill* by Dr. Jolene Brighten is an excellent resource; she also shares her knowledge in a number of podcasts easily found online.

While there are myriad teachings about supporting your cycle and reproductive potential, the first thing to grasp is the very simple overview. Nutritious, balanced eating, great sleep, a calm state of mind, and as natural a lifestyle as possible are what this incredible orchestration of signals and surges requires to work well. As Lauren told us, a balanced, harmonious menstrual cycle will typically be the outcome when you live a lifestyle that preserves the jing. Oh, and one more thing. Wear socks! Really. The Chinese aunties in us cringe at seeing a woman's bare feet gracing cold floors, because, as Lauren points out, the energy channels for the Kidney, Liver, and Spleen start at the feet! A chill at the toes can cause constriction and stagnation of chi in these three highways of reproductive energy. Unless it's tropical or a heatwave is striking, always keep your feet toasty.

release your stress

As soft gray light filters in through the windows of an airy apartment in London, England, the Vedic wellness expert and meditation instructor Jillian Lavender guides a group of women in a simple seated practice that slows their heart rate, relaxes their vascular system, and allows tension to release like pressure from a valve. Though the women's eyes are closed, Jillian can see frown lines begin to soften and the rise and fall of their breath become freer, less constricted. In the twenty minutes they sit comfortably, practicing the effortless technique of Vedic meditation, their parasympathetic (or rest-and-digest) nervous system takes the reins inside, helping to create conditions in the body that wash away the residues of stress. Shoulders melt, and so do facades, as the technique draws them inward toward stillness.

For all these women whose plates are crowded with personal and professional demands, daily meditation will become as nonnegotiable as brushing their teeth, a foundation of their health and wellness. But this is particularly true of those planning to start a family. Physiological stress responses, teaches Jillian, are the biggest cause of disharmony in a woman's reproductive center.

evaluating your starting point

NO MATTER how up close and personal you get with your period, there are basic health parameters to check into before getting closer to conception that go beyond well-woman checkups and Pap tests. Consider the following seven basic parameters of well-being, then ask your partner to do similarly, for several of them apply equally to him.

Weight: Being over or under your body's healthiest weight can have significant effects on ovulation.

Blood sugar: Dysglycemia (abnormally high or low blood sugar) can be disruptive to fertility and contribute to low thyroid function.

Vitamin D_3 levels: A critical driver of so many bodily activities, including fertility, this is important and easy to check as part of routine bloodwork or via tests ordered online. If you're low (most people are), start to turn it around with daily supplementation and sun exposure, then track it. Seek a supplement combining vitamins D_3 and K_2. Two thousand IUs is a good starting dose for most (unless you have the autoimmune condition sarcoidosis), but if you are very low, consult with your provider about a higher dose. We love the sun-exposure app D Minder.

Thyroid function: Your supersensitive thyroid gland, wrapping around your windpipe like a butterfly, helps you make hormones, but it is highly susceptible to pollution, stress, and nutritional lacks. Give it some love. Check your temperature when you awaken in the morning (aka your basal body temperature) using the specific technique taught in the FAM method, and if it is consistently below 97°F (36.1°C), pledge to do some investigating. (The next step would be talking to your health practitioner about doing comprehensive thyroid blood panels to check your status.) Good thyroid health does not only help a woman become and stay pregnant; experts now say a baby's neurological development can be hampered by low thyroid function in both parents, and even subtle dips in thyroid levels warrant attention. Read up on functional medicine approaches (a quick internet search will deliver volumes of info; Dr. Datis Kharrazian is a trusted expert) to get the lowdown on proper testing and protecting your thyroid.

Gut health: Experiencing any festering gut issues like candida, leaky gut, or SIBO (small intestinal bacterial overgrowth)? Now's the time to methodically clear it out, ideally with the support of an experienced practitioner; you need a healthy gut to properly absorb nutrients and alleviate systemic stress.

Autoimmune issues: Wise one and ancestral nutrition expert Nora Gedgaudas told us her wish for all women pre-pregnancy would be to screen for any potential undiagnosed autoimmune conditions and/or potential triggers, especially dietary intolerances (her gold-standard tests are from Cyrex Laboratories). She says that diagnosed and undiagnosed maternal autoimmunity can be a vector in autism and other immunological vulnerabilities in your unborn child. (Gedgaudas says Hashimoto's thyroiditis is one of the most common autoimmune conditions in women.) Following dedicated dietary discipline (which Nora says should be rich in the highest quality animal-source proteins, fats, fat-soluble vitamins, and essential fatty acids), cleansing, and gut-repair protocols can achieve tremendous turnarounds, especially when you catch an autoimmune issue early. If you know or suspect you are a candidate for A-I repair, the prelude to pregnancy is a golden opportunity to address this with a slow and steady protocol of healing care.

Teeth: Make that dental appointment you've been blowing off! Pregnancy can make gums and teeth become looser and more vulnerable, and make your mouth more susceptible to bacterial growth.

Bonus tip: Testing for a mutation of the MTHFR gene is an advanced step typically performed after difficulty maintaining a pregnancy, but finding out this information earlier in your health journey can be priceless. (One clue you may be a candidate for testing is a history of depression or migraines; others can easily be discovered online.) Knowing your MTHFR status can help you customize your diet and supplement regimen in advance with the support of a practitioner well versed in this issue—especially in regard to folate supplementation and methylation support—to help you sustain a viable and healthy pregnancy. At-home tests are available, though due to the nuances of this subject, it's wise to enlist expert help. ○

That's largely due to the play of the stress hormones adrenaline and cortisol, which are released when the nervous system perceives a situation to be urgent, anxiety-inducing, or downright dangerous, and the aftereffects they cause. (Her interest is personal: she conceived her daughter at age forty-five and attributes her success to Vedic meditation along with Ayurvedic panchakarma and lifestyle protocols.)

If you were to see a Chinese medicine or Ayurvedic practitioner after dealing with ongoing stress—which would make you the norm, not the exception today—they may not use these Western terms. But the general understanding is the same. Stress response in the body disrupts *everything*, from the ability to digest and absorb nutrients and detoxify, to the capacity to hang on to your jing or your ojas—your super-subtle life-giving reserves. Remember the all-important Kidney organ system—the place your adrenal glands reside? The jolts and shocks of everyday stress deplete it something fierce, because an adrenaline rush is your first-line response to stressors of all kinds—physical, mental, and emotional. This depletion might manifest first as a Kidney yang deficiency, the inability to transform jing into hormones and other physiological functions; if uncorrected, it can become a Kidney yin deficiency, a weakness in the maintaining and repairing functions of the body. You can reframe this in another vernacular: overwork the adrenals and their sister stress hormone cortisol, and a domino effect begins. Your body, seeking help from *somewhere*, starts to draw energy from the thyroid, tiring it out; then it can turn to the hormones that govern your weight and blood sugar, destabilizing those, and then to the sex hormones. Everywhere the dominoes touch, wear and tear ensues.

A brief look at cortisol is key here, because where adrenaline disperses fairly quickly, cortisol hangs around for a day or two after it's emitted. It's like a social media influencer—it shows up constantly, has a wide reach, and can get a little aggravating. Let's not give cortisol a bad rap, though! Cortisol is supposed to rise and fall in sync with your wake/sleep cycles. This very yang hormone is motivating and stimulating and helps you have steady energy, a good mood, stable blood sugar, and good sleep. But when it gets out of balance, spiking throughout the day in response to situations that either consciously or unconsciously are *freaking you out*, super yang cortisol can cause long-lasting disruption in your body. The most obvious problem when it comes to preconception? Too much cortisol in your system communicates the news that your body is under fire and underresourced, and not currently a safe or supported place for pregnancy to occur. Your sensitive sex hormones, which exist to support your body to create new life successfully, get the message to press pause on regular programming—and a disrupted cycle can be the result. You only have so much energy on board, and in the hierarchy of biology, survival trumps reproduction, and energy and nutrients are diverted to cortisol production at the expense of proper progesterone and thyroid hormone production.

Here's a simple way to look at stress and reproduction. Where sex hormones build things up, stress hormones break things down. If you let your stress response spike and spike again without taking action to turn it around, slowly, you might feel depressed or disinterested in sex—a hint that libido-pumping testosterone has taken a dive. (Both women and men have testosterone; men just have more of it.) You might have digestive issues, put on weight you can't shake, sleep poorly, and feel tired all the time, or be tired-and-wired, a sign of screwy cortisol levels no longer following natural ebbs and flows. Inadvertently, you can tire out adrenals further by relying on caffeine to compensate—a habit the herbalist Chad Cornell says "burns through your jing and steals from your older self." And, no surprise here, the delicate interplay of estrogen and progesterone can get wobbly. Ovulation can be delayed, the luteal phase can shorten—now it's harder for a fertilized egg to successfully implant—and circulation can be affected, too. During a stress response, blood flow diverts to your extremities; this steals blood and warmth away from your reproductive organs, potentially messing up ovulation and the warming that naturally happens after.

You probably can't control the amount of demands and stressors you face daily. Opting out of solving problems, handling conflicts, and avoiding other people's road rage is likely not an option. What you *can* do is train your nervous system to respond to challenging situations differently, which will reduce the stress surges and avoid the damaging domino effect. A weird

When you're under stress, don't forget the obvious: touch! Show your partner your system needs a little loving. Invite fingertips to trace your skin. Give yourself a massage or enjoy a sensual moment. Touch is the ultimate oxytocin enhancer.

thing happens when stress responses pile up. You become hypervigilant, trip-wired to surge with stress hormones at the smallest trigger. That's your body telling you it feels pushed to last-resort measures. (If your glands could speak, they'd yell, *I've got no way to deal with this event, I'm deploying my emergency chute!*) Jillian says that's a misperception of a nervous system that's been pushed too far. Rationally speaking, you likely *could* deal with the deadline or the parking ticket. But the reserve tank of energy you draw upon to adapt to unexpected events, to pivot when plans change, or to push through a tough moment is empty. Added to that, the stress response has become so normalized, it's as if the body can barely remember how to go the opposite way and sink down from stimulating yang into the slower and quieter yin state that fills those reserve tanks like water from a well. Jillian, like every wise one we spoke with, emphasized that inserting daily habits that actively "switch on" the latter state of restoration is key. It's not enough to just *think* about being less stressed or to stick a "Don't stress!" note on your mirror; you want to *create* the anti-stress state in your physiology, to show your body the pathway down.

There are lots of ways to do this. Conscious breathing, the ultimate anywhere-anytime stress-busting tool, lowers stress chemistry immediately. Long, slow breaths that engage the diaphragm activate the parasympathetic nervous system and send a helpful message body-wide: *I'm safe!* Stretching and breathing together (namaste, yoga!) increases the effect more. Yogic postures gently massage the organs and the glands, unwind muscular tension patterns, and move energy where it's gotten stuck. To simplify greatly, this teaches your body to adopt a physiology of calm. (Try Yin Yoga—it's bliss.) Tai chi and qigong help you "exercise your insides," as some teachers say, restoring whole-system balance through calming movements. Listening to binaural

TREAT YOUR SYSTEM TO PEACE

- *Spend three to five minutes sitting quietly,* doing nothing, before starting your day.

- *Move in any way you enjoy.* Exercise flushes cortisol from the bloodstream and floods you with mood-boosting chemicals.

- *Write.* Journaling and reflecting for a few moments at the start or end of your day lets you leave worries on the page. Do it by hand— it slows down thoughts and heart rate.

- *Say "No, thanks"* to invitations and opportunities that take more energy than they give.

- *Get enough sleep.* When you're not well rested, you more quickly tip into stress.

- *Have sex!* All kinds of oxytocin-promoting touching help, in particular deep orgasms.

- *Treat yourself* to acupuncture, chiropractic care, or a *sobada* abdominal massage. Releasing tension energetically and physically helps your body return to homeostasis. Acupuncture can help direct greater blood flow toward the ovaries and uterus, helping with cycle regulation and fertility, as well as rebalance stressed sex hormones and improve ovarian function and egg production.

beats, walking barefoot in nature, or swimming in the ocean can also reset your mental and physical state. The hormone specialist Sara Gottfried, MD, teaches that men are wired to respond to stress with "fight or flight," but women are wired differently; our nervous system drives us to "tend and befriend," seeking experiences that will raise our love and bonding hormone, oxytocin, in order to settle our system. (Oxytocin is extremely health-boosting physically as well as mentally-emotionally.) Sometimes that longing can drive us to things that inadvertently make it worse. Gottfried says that alcohol and sugar actually raise cortisol. (A healthful salty snack, by contrast, can raise oxytocin—try some miso-avocado toast or cream cheese dotted with soy sauce on salty crackers!) Connecting with others, turning toward them to feel safer and more supported is our nature. An intimate get-together with a friend, a group movement class, or a women's circle in which support is freely given and received not only feels good; it literally changes the chemistry in your body, improving stress *and*

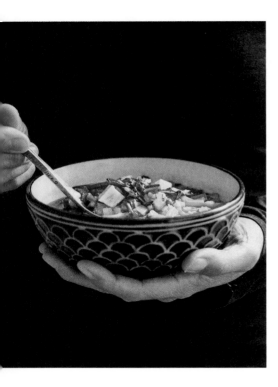

sex hormones, and as the old ways say, increasing your ojas (some even correlate that substance with oxytocin). Laughter while doing any of those things: extra credit.

But the motherlode of anti-stress practices has to be meditation. Because meditation techniques exist to deliberately open a door to a different state in the brain and the body, committing to a daily practice is like staging an intervention on a stressed nervous system, taking it by the shoulders and showing it another way to be. Your body gets the actual experience of settling and quieting when you meditate, and by repeating this consistently, it remembers what it forgot. *Oh, yes,* says your heart, and your blood pressure, and your hormones, *calm! I like how this feels!* You've likely heard how when you sleep, your physiology naturally restores and heals. Daytime meditation is a super bonus round of resting when deep refills of energy can occur.

Sometimes—but not always—the reduction of physical activity draws the mind down, too, relieving it of engaging in all those pesky recirculating thoughts and concerns. After a while, your mind learns there's more space

If you don't yet have a meditation practice, Jillian recommends this simple exercise to help the body settle down and begin to release stress and tension:

- Sit easily, close the eyes, and take a moment to get comfortable.

- Bring your attention to sensations in the body.

- Somewhere in the body there will be a dominant sensation. It can be anything—tightness in the chest; a tingle on top of the head; even an itch on the big left toe.

- Gently bring attention to the sensation. There is no need to concentrate or focus; simply let the attention lightly rest there.

- After a moment, that sensation will shift and dissolve, and another sensation will become primary.

- Let the attention move to this new sensation and locale in the body—a twinge in the hip from yesterday's exercise; a tightness in the back of the neck; or a feeling of lightness in the stomach.

- Again, after a few moments, this will begin to dissipate and another part of the body will draw your attention. Continue in the same way.

- After just a few minutes, you'll naturally find yourself thinking other thoughts easily—almost a sensation of daydreaming. Open the eyes slowly.

available than it realized and it doesn't have to feel pushed into a tight corner, reactive and antsy. Meditation can feel wonderful, and equally, it can sometimes feel mundane. But if you stick with it, you discover its benefits off the meditation chair (or couch, or car seat, or wherever you have time to do it). By resting and restoring in daily micro-chunks, your body develops a greater capacity to respond to demands without deploying emergency adrenaline. Consequently, your nervous system stops seeing everything as a stress, and as a result, your mind learns it can move through challenges successfully and find solutions in all that extra space. It doesn't have to be so scared. You create a *positive* domino effect, building better well-being instead of creating collateral damage. A good reason to adopt the habit now? The less stress chemistry in your body when pregnant, the less you pass on to baby, protecting their health and even their IQ and cognition skills.

Whichever method of meditation you choose, it's safe to say that this practice of seemingly doing nothing actually does everything, helping body and mind find their way to the state of balance and harmony that nurturing new life depends on.

create a lower-tox lifestyle

In the shadow of Colorado's Rocky Mountains, Dr. Sarah Villafranco tests her company's newest skin-nourishing and all-natural body oil, free of sketchy ingredients like parabens and phthalates. This former ER doc and mother of two daughters founded her aromatherapeutic beauty brand Osmia Organics to help women walk away from products that contain hormone-scrambling chemicals. Attuned to the cascades of inflammation, free radical damage, and reproductive issues that can occur from cumulative exposure to toxins, Sarah wants to normalize a lifestyle where everything rubbed, slathered, and sprayed on a woman's body, and even used in her home, is safe. Ditto, obviously, for her masculine mate—pollutants can damage a man's sperm motility and concentration just like they can disrupt your cycle and negatively affect your eggs. Experts say they're a major cause of the decline in sperm health over the past seventy years.

Sarah knows that umbilical cords transfer the body burden of chemicals and pollutants from mother to child and that modern women's breastmilk typically contains dangerous industrial chemicals such as perfluorinated compounds and metals such as mercury. She can quote studies showing that women with detectable levels of parabens in their urine can have significantly shorter menstrual cycles, potentially disrupting ovulation and implantation. She can also explain why the busier the liver gets detoxifying environmental toxins, the less effectively it can help balance your hormones. But she doesn't trade in fear tactics. Sarah's personal mantra is "Stop fighting, start inviting." It means, proceed with excitement, not anxiety. Put your focus not on all the dangers that lurk in every shadow, but rather on the fresh and positive things you can invite into your life: a naturally scented body oil made only from a cocktail of plant oils that feels delicious on naked skin; a mineral-based sunscreen that's ocean-safe, too; a hip new menstrual underwear product that replaces an old-school chemically bleached tampon. It's okay to take this one change at a time. Because fairly quickly, these choices start to crowd out the harmful ones until your landscape looks quite different. On the way you might feel inspired and uplifted, too, more in touch with your body and senses. It's no longer hippie or out-there to connect the dots between everyday chemicals, measurable endocrine disruption, and dysfunction or disease; it's scientifically validated common sense.

It's naïve to pretend that a clean sweep of every potentially harmful product can happen overnight, or that it doesn't sometimes cost more at first (until you learn to hack the system by making DIY things like green home cleaners, a remarkably simple task). But know that the more ways you can reduce environmental toxins from the everyday lives of you and your mate, the more relief you give your body from fertility-impairing inflammation, endocrine disruption, and the stress of handling toxins. (Toxic chemicals, metals, and radiation can also damage DNA of eggs and sperm and negatively impact gene expression.) There's a reason that today's burgeoning category of essential oil brands have found their biggest advocates in mothers: making the switch to a total green, clean routine is one of the best things you can do for your reproductive health and that of your future child. (Not only in utero; you'll want a chemical-free environment once he's born.)

As you spend time in this Preparing phase, take a good look around the places you live and work in daily. What do I put on, in, and around my body that I'm not quite sure about? Is it *actually* safe? Do some detective work. Read the labels and start to research online. Today, it's not hard. The Environmental Working Group (ewg.org) is a good place to begin, and "clean beauty" and "green home" topics are now covered in mainstream news. Be a skeptic; be a weirdo if you need to be, insisting on bringing your own water containers to work. Here are the seven areas to look at as you ready your field for planting:

WHAT YOU EAT: You've heard it before, but it bears repeating. Reduce foods grown with pesticides, herbicides, and fungicides to the barest minimum. Make it a mission to seek organic produce, grains, pantry products, and dairy you can afford. Online healthy grocery vendors, co-ops, and food-buying clubs are making this easier. Pledge to avoid GMO crops grown using the herbicide glyphosate, a known carcinogen and fertility disruptor. Spend some time critiquing your meat and eggs—what feed or drugs were fed to these animals? (Toxins bioaccumulate; they increase up the food chain.) Cut down on canned ingredients (can linings contain BPA) and plastic storage materials (switch to glass containers), and *never* heat foods in plastic in the microwave. And plastic water bottles? Old school. Go glass or stainless steel. Ditch the aluminum foil for cooking your food and use beeswax wraps. While you're looking around your kitchen, keep an eye out for nonstick cooking pans. The chemicals used to coat conventional nonstick pans are highly toxic, especially when they get chipped from use. Consider replacing them with ceramic-coated nonstick pans or use stainless steel or ceramic pans whenever possible.

WHAT YOU DRINK: We're talking water here. Explore the best level of water filter you can afford and make a splash. Tap water contains traces of unwanted metals

> Most people don't dive into healthier skin and personal care until they have a fear-based reason to do so. It's a pity, because they could be diving in way sooner, enjoying gorgeous, natural products that enhance physical and mental well-being in ways conventional products can't even approach.
>
> —SARAH VILLAFRANCO, MD
> founder of Osmia Organics

and chemicals, which cause toxicity and displace other minerals, as well as hormone-disrupting pharmaceuticals, like the residues of *other* women's birth control pills. (EWG.org has a water filter guide.) Your skin "drinks up" tons of water when you shower or bathe, too, so don't forget a filter in the bathroom; they need not cost a lot and are quite easy to install.

WHAT YOU APPLY: Audit your regularly used self-care products, going head to toe: from hair color to teeth cleaners (and whiteners!), from lashes to lips, from underarms to nails, from the fragrances that get dabbed right onto your neck's lymph nodes to beauty interventions like Botox and fillers. And don't forget those tampons or chlorine-bleached pads. How many things do you apply or use daily that potentially infuse industrial chemicals into your body, via your skin or internal membranes? The total body burden may be more than you realize. If you aren't ready to go 100 percent body-friendly (yet), what deals will you make to lighten the total load? You can't live without that red lip color? Trade in the aluminum-based deodorant to help pay its biological tax. You can't throw a rock without hitting an innovative clean beauty brand today. This won't be hard.

WHAT YOU USE TO CLEAN: As above, not difficult. Healthy, low-tox cleaning products abound. Essential oil cleaning recipes proliferate. (Mix, shake, spray.) Educate yourself about the hidden risks in stuff you might overlook: detergents, room fresheners, dryer sheets. And remember that thing called fresh air? Open a window! Hang your sheets on a line. Find a safe or green dry cleaner if you need one. What you particularly *don't* want is to inhale all that nasty industrial cleaning stuff with windows closed, nor any off-gassing from furnishings you live or work amid.

WHAT YOU USE TO RELAX: Okay, this one's not about synthetic chemicals, but while you're doing that audit . . . nix the tobacco (duh), and if you use marijuana cannabis of any kind, give it a rest at the very least during the three-month ramp-up to conceiving. This is especially applicable to men, because marijuana cannabis and energetic, robust sperm don't go together, but its use can affect female fertility, too. And don't be tempted to fall back on alcohol as a relaxant! More than one daily drink can affect sperm production in men, and alcohol raises women's estrogen, disrupting our natural balance (one drink can raise it anywhere from 11 to 15 percent). As for hot baths and saunas? Excessive heat can also hinder sperm vitality (and can even cause disruptive levels of heat within you!). Dial it down—save the super-hot baths for later!

WHAT ILLUMINATES YOUR FIELD: What's the one nutrient we consume all day, and increasingly, much of the night as well, that we rarely think about? Light. Light can be considered a significant nutrient that tells your body what to do and when to do it. Your cells work *with* it constantly. For example, morning sunlight on your eyes and skin sets you up to make proper amounts of melatonin, a hormone that helps regulate rhythms of sleep, appetite, and menstruation, among many other things. Sleeping in true dark at night does the next step, ensuring the pituitary actually secretes good amounts of melatonin. Sounds simple enough, except that we don't get enough true dark. We light up our lives after sunset with sun-mimicking white light bulbs and ever-present blue-light screens that do a number on natural melatonin production. Not only does sleep and hormone balance take a hit, but your liver's detoxifying work gets hampered because it too works in sync with rhythms of light and dark.

You have a few choices: turn off technology after sunset, install effective blue light–filtering software like Iris on your computer (this book's writers use it religiously—get it at iristech.co), or wear blue light–blocking glasses. You can even install amber light bulbs quite easily at home—this lets you avoid blue light–emitting LEDs. Whichever way you go, be sure your bedroom is always pitch black! Blackening your bedroom completely can even be the switch that gets an irregular menstrual cycle on track—it's that powerful. And during the day, get sun on your skin (safely!). You want to build up that vitamin D.

ONE LAST THING . . . Reduce your exposure to nonnative EMFs wherever you can. EMFs are the electromagnetic fields emitted by devices and wireless technology. They're hard to dodge, impossible to see, yet exert an insidious stress on your cellular functioning and reproductive potential. Turn your router off at night when your resting nervous system is more vulnerable to EMFs, keep your cell phone away from your body and use it less frequently (men *must* keep them away from their groins!), never place your laptop on your lap either before or during pregnancy (or ever, basically), and get smart about other high EMF-emitters that may be on or just around your home (smart meters, cell antennae, cell towers, and so on). Your body's biofield will thank you for it.

give your liver some love

Taxicab horns honk on busy streets below the quiet treatment room where Dr. Linda Lancaster meets her New York City clientele. The naturopath, homeopath, and energy medicine healer is the epitome of a wise woman elder; with her hair streaked with silvery gray, decades of yogic service to her name, and having circumnavigated the globe endless times on her healing journey, she truly has seen it all. Where would this titan of subtle medicine start should you consult her about readying your body for pregnancy? Your liver. This organ is a star player in digestion and the epicenter of detoxification, and even though it sits above and over from your reproductive organs (under your right rib cage, to be exact), it exerts considerable influence on your vitality, resiliency, and hormone balance—the conditions for preconception. But it's also vulnerable, and Dr. Linda, as her patients call her, says that almost everyone she treats has a tired, overworked liver that needs some deliberate care.

It's not surprising! Your liver works multiple jobs at once. As the epicenter of your digestive "fire," as the old ways describe it, the liver helps to digest or break down foods into components your body can absorb and use, and even synthesizes cholesterol to make new hormones and vitamin D. It also metabolizes or takes apart old, used-up estrogen hormones so they *don't* get reabsorbed and disrupt your estrogen/progesterone balance. It does the same for damaging toxins that have been absorbed, inhaled, or consumed from your environment, your diet, and your everyday products, pills, and potions, breaking them down into forms that can be excreted so that they don't disrupt your hormones and threaten your health.

strong mom

WISE ONE and pregnancy and postpartum athleticism coach Brianna Battles advocates getting in shape well in advance of pregnancy. She says that building strength in your body through your favorite form of resistance training tremendously affects your mental, emotional, *and* physical health, giving you a level of adaptability that helps you live comfortably and empowered in your changing body, more resilient to ups and downs that may occur. She also advocates basic anatomical awareness: learning how your diaphragm and pelvic floor work together, how to feel into your abdominal wall and the tension you tend to hold there. Women unconsciously suck in their tummies all day or constrict their breath, which causes the pelvic floor muscles to tighten in a kind of grip. Add the weight of a baby on top, and the pressure can create problems. Brianna is passionate about teaching women to manage and improve some very common postpartum dysfunctions like incontinence, lower back pain, diastasis recti—a condition that occurs when the gap in your rectus abdominus muscles caused by your expanding abdomen does not close normally after delivery—and pelvic organ prolapse. (Many of these things can be exacerbated by incorrect exercising in postpartum, too.) Whether you work out regularly or not (yet), she advocates a prehab approach: take some time to connect to your body from the inside out to avoid ever getting to a "wish someone had told me" moment after birth. A skilled coach trained in Brianna's methods can help build this awareness, as can a pelvic floor physical therapist—Brianna says one session in advance of pregnancy can make a world of difference down the line. ⬡

Your liver also performs another undercelebrated function: it ensures your bowels keep moving by assisting the gallbladder in making bile, a substance that both breaks down fats for use in the body and sweeps unwanted hormones and toxins out through the colon. This is more critical than it may seem, because chronic constipation can affect hormone balance and can put pressure on the reproductive organs, hindering their easeful function. Constipation is a super-common condition today that exerts a much greater impact on reproduction than we realize, says wise one Marcia Lopez, so addressing it should be a priority in the preconception months. The liver does even more than this, too, like storing essential vitamins and minerals—micronutrients you'll need during pregnancy—like a master bank vault full of items of great value. Dr. Linda says the liver also metabolizes the thoughts you think and the emotions you feel; it's the master processor for your body, mind, and spirit.

We could go on. But you probably get the picture. You want your liver in tip-top shape as you prepare your field and as you build your soil. It's your ally, and when it's out of balance, such as when it gets overloaded with toxins, or slowed down by congesting foods, your reproductive health can be as well.

How does a woman without training in, say, herbal medicine or acupressure, give her liver some TLC? Simple: she reduces the burden she puts on it, and she feeds it foods that give it a boost. The first stress on your liver comes from diet, says Dr. Linda. Certain foods congest it, causing its function to slow. Highly processed and junk foods are no-brainers—they contain congesting ingredients *and* chemicals, a double whammy on the liver. Ditto lots of alcohol and caffeine. Both require metabolizing before they can be excreted. But foods to audit include things that may surprise you, like refined and overly heated vegetable oils, heavy and dense baked goods, and excessive nuts and dairy. Dr. Linda even advises caution with coconut, a drupe (stone fruit) and not technically a nut, but heavy and clogging to the liver if you go wild with it, especially as an oil or a cream.

The second stress on the liver comes from processing the pollution that's part of contemporary life. Chemicals and metals in the air, water, and food, in medications and personal-care products, even in your mouth fillings, if unchecked, can accumulate and disrupt all kinds of functioning, from top to bottom, in your body (not to mention a baby's). As your primary detoxification organ, the liver does its best to clear unwanted contaminants from your bloodstream, but with all that it faces today, the burden to detoxify is great.

The third stress is mental and emotional: both repressed anger and frustration are the cause of liver "stagnation," the Chinese medicine word for congested energy in this organ system; a sluggish, low-functioning liver can also *cause* these states, as its fire starts to rage unbalanced, causing excessive heat. The heat can manifest in many ways, not just as outbursts and irritation, but also as headaches.

Reducing all three of these categories of stress the best you can helps your liver do its job. But that's not always enough. Once you take some of those challenging inputs away, the space remains for alternatives that help this organ do its work. Dark leafy greens, vegetables with a bitter taste such as asparagus, artichoke, and superbitter dandelion, as well as cruciferous vegetables are manna to the liver, keeping it clear; compounds in these foods support its two detoxifying phases. Likewise, beets, filled with mesmerizing red pigments, are a humble superfood that help your liver purify your blood. Astringent citrus fruits such as lemon and grapefruit help to clear congestion and rev up its function, along with plenty of clean, filtered water, and sour tastes of all kinds soothe it. Unheated extra-virgin olive oil is a balm to the liver and gallbladder, and turmeric is its bright-golden friend. Plants such as milk thistle, burdock, and oregano keep it in balance.

Dr. Linda suggests that women at all phases of their lives, and naturally, men, too, perform a biannual or even seasonal gentle liver-cleansing diet for twenty-one days to give this vital organ a real break. (This carries extra *oomph* if you've been on hormonal birth control for years; your liver could use support after processing those pharmaceuticals!) The methodology she outlines in her book *Harmonic Healing* (written with our cowriter Amely) is inexpensive and food-based, using recipes such as Ayurvedic kitchari, green soups, bone broths, and refreshingly sour morning smoothies. (Many of the natural ingredients used also create conditions where an irritated gut lining can begin to heal.) It even includes naturopathic baths for reducing the effect of environmental pollutants and dry brushing for lymphatic stimulation. Together, these things will help your liver get back up to speed if it's become sluggish, and soothed if it's inflamed, so it can help keep your estrogen levels in check and your reserves of nutrition high.

There are other ways to clean house, though. Traditional Ayurvedic panchakarma treatments use very simple foods, and often lots of gut-soothing ghee, to clear ama and balance excess of doshas. Functional medicine cleanses, meanwhile, reboot total gastrointestinal health while promoting heightened detoxification using specialty supplements and, often, accoutrements like infrared saunas. By working with a professional trained in functional medicine, you might ramp up the cleansing further if you have the means, by testing your hair or your blood for metals, and if they're high, creating a program to gradually reduce them. This can become as tailored as you can afford and can include genetic testing to see how your body detoxifies and how your unique hormone balance is affected as a result. Please note that metal-clearing programs should be performed at least six months before potential pregnancy to ensure no metals are circulating in your system.

Not sure you have the mojo to take on an actual period of dedicated cleansing like this? Your everyday lifestyle can still be super effective! When you remove excess alcohol and poor-quality foods, go big on the roughage, including bitter vegetables and beets, drink digestion-soothing broth, and have touches of sour in your diet, this entire way of feeding yourself will show your liver tremendous love and will ripple out to smoother functioning in your reproductive organs and menstrual cycle. Good news: this is exactly the approach to eating shared in Chapter 5, Fortifying! The commonality among all these approaches to caring for the fire of digestion and the power of detoxification is that they feed the body while rejuvenating it, which tends to be wiser than fasting-type cleanses—especially if you're doing this in cooler months, harsher climates, or have a body type that doesn't handle long periods without solid food well.

chapter

4

clearing

In a small town in southern Germany, in a quaint building on a quiet street, is a candle-lit room. Here a healer softly chants a series of Sanskrit words, called a bija mantra, while a woman rests on a mat absorbing the soothing sounds. This healer, Ulrike Remlein, works with women at all stages of life and holds a special place for mothers-to-be and their partners, supporting them along the journey to conception, through pregnancy, and into the raw and wild early days of motherhood. At the heart of her work is the heart of creation: the womb. If you work with Ulrike you will be gently but firmly guided to connect with the source of a woman's power and creative potential, which rests in this often ignored region of the body.

The uterus is the first home of every
human on the planet and therefore it
is important that we take care of it!

—MARCIA LOPEZ,
holistic reproductive wellness practitioner

While you likely have an awareness of your womb—you know it's where babies take up residence for nine and a half months—you may not see it as a gateway into greater empowerment and freedom. That's because, in a sense, your womb has been napping. Ulrike calls her work "womb awakening." It's a process of personal discovery that begins with a recognition that you came preinstalled with a powerful energy center that plays a key role in creating life *and* in supporting your own growth and development. Connecting to your womb helps you recognize, and heal, parts of yourself that have been lost or buried deep. Womb awakening is a remembering of who you really are. The womb is our creative center and power center, Ulrike reminds her clients. Without an awakened womb it is really hard to create anything beautiful—or create anything at all.

What better metaphor for the circle of life, the holder of interconnecting and opposing yin and yang, do we have in our body than the womb? This epicenter in a woman's body is the ultimate source of output and creation (yang, all the way) and it's also where she holds unprocessed emotion (a decidedly yin factor). These emotions are often connected to identity and self-esteem, motherhood, birth, and sexuality. And when they are unaddressed, they can take up space and energy and can interfere with what you hope to bring into your life, whether it's a baby, a new job, a life partner, or another dream. It's just human nature: Once unwanted things get shelved out of sight, they tend to sit in storage for years. Emotional pain can be hard to face, downright scary. But it's worth tapping the courage to turn the lock, turn on the light, and take a look, for if you have experienced any level of trauma—impossible to escape in a lifetime—and not acknowledged it, you will be trailed by an echo that will continue to reverberate into your present life. As Ulrike likes to say, the challenging emotions must be seen, felt, and released so you don't drown in their energy and so you can shine fully.

Why the womb? As this residue of unaddressed emotion accumulates it needs a place to reside in the body. It could inhabit your lower back or your shoulders—they're certainly achy enough—but the deepest emotional hurts and traumas are tucked away in your womb, the perfect, dark storehouse for these challenging currents of energy. Women who are more attuned to the workings of nuanced energies say they can sense blocks to the energy around this area of the body, but most of us are disconnected from the subtle language of the womb. And though it may seem strange, tuning into your womb is an extremely worthy endeavor. Experts think so, too. The wise ones say that if a woman hopes to access the power of the womb, and the potential for creating life that it holds, there must first be a reckoning with what is stored there.

This reckoning or acknowledgment is an essential aspect of pre-pregnancy preparation, as important as breaking harmful habits like smoking or excessive drinking. Recognizing, and then releasing, the emotions stored in your womb is a process we call *clearing*. Clearing is about addressing what is unspoken and unresolved, not about removing or fixing pieces of yourself. It's an invitation to

STUCK EMOTIONS

We learn to repress what is not welcome. Those emotions get stuck in our body, they become cellular memories; they are stored as body sensations and emotions, feelings and blockages in the body, and can even make you physically sick if you don't deal with the emotions. The deepest repressed stuff we store in the womb; that is the place where the deepest emotions live.

—ULRIKE REMLEIN, *womb awakening mentor and red tent facilitator* get to know all the layers of who you are, gently exploring the parts deep inside, like a revealing of the mini figurines tucked inside a Russian doll.

Pregnancy preparation is a time to take inventory of yourself at every level: physically, emotionally, and spiritually, and Clearing is a path to reconnecting to the parts of yourself that have been lost or buried deep. This is a remembering of who you really are and a reclaiming of the pieces of yourself that have been left behind. In many shamanic traditions, those seeking true spiritual liberation are instructed to journey within themselves to collect the versions of themselves that fractured off after experiencing pain or trauma. This is accomplished by turning toward the hurt that you felt, and that still resides in you, acknowledging it, and then letting it go—a process that's similar to caring for in injured bird, helping it heal, and then sending it back into the world. Giving this level of tenderness and attention to your own hurts will help you come back to wholeness, making you a stronger and more viable foundation for conception, pregnancy, motherhood, and beyond.

We're the first to admit that this level of emotional work can make the more clinical aspects of preparing for pregnancy look downright fun. Eliminating caffeine and junk food, following a stress management protocol, and exercising more can seem like a cake walk compared with facing the parts of yourself that have been pushed into the dark corners of your being. Ironically, this can be especially true if you're already walking the path of self-awareness.

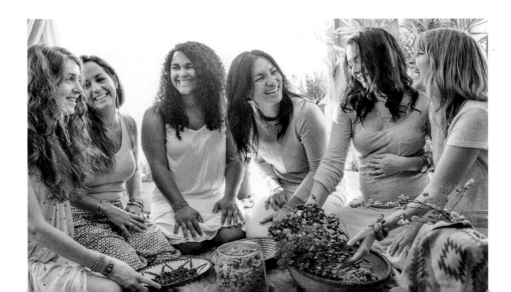

So often meditation and energy practices take us blissfully upward to lighter realms—there's that upward-moving prana vata again—that we can forget, or avoid, the downward energy or the "lower chakras where the energy tends to be challenging," as Ulrike says. As we've learned, however, riding that downward-moving apana vata is important, too, for the lower energy centers and lower parts of the body must not be ignored. But getting to know yourself in a more honest way doesn't have to be scary or disruptive. It can look as simple as spending time connecting to your womb (don't worry, we'll show you how later in this chapter) and noting the messages or information that you receive when you focus there, or as in-depth as a full exploration of past traumas. The degree to which you dive into what is held in your womb is up to you. If you discover that hard emotions

When the womb is honored and respected, she becomes a channel of power, creativity, and beauty—and joy reigns on earth. When her voice goes unheard, unanswered, denied, the womb becomes a vessel of disease. . . . The condition of women's wombs also directly reflects the condition of women's minds, spirits, and actions. The womb is a storehouse of all our emotions. It collects every feeling—good and bad.

—FROM *SACRED WOMAN*,
QUEEN AFUA

are coming up as you experiment with the practices in this chapter, please seek outside help. You don't have to do it alone (and you shouldn't try to). Turn to your partner, a trusted friend, a therapist, or one of the wise ones listed on page 16.

Many indigenous traditions have always recognized the power of the womb, understanding that it is a woman's source of power and the mighty creator of life, but the modern woman's interest in this area of herself is fairly recent. Buoyed by vociferous Instagrammers reclaiming lost wisdom and celebrating sisterhood, the womb is beginning to garner some overdue attention. It has the heart to thank. As more women wake up to the fact that they have become slaves to their mind, getting continually tossed around by its onslaught

THE RITE OF THE WOMB

Rosalba Fontanez is a Mexican initiate in a Quechua-Peruvian Shamanic lineage. She works with women on the path to pregnancy, supporting their spiritual healing as they prepare to walk through the gate to motherhood. She guides women through thirteen rites to facilitate this transformation. In the Rite of the Womb, she has the woman recite a specific mantra to her womb and to her mother's womb. The words she directs to her womb, and to her mother's, state a clear intention: this essential part of her being is not a place to store fear or pain; rather, it's a place to create and hold light. The words she repeats are powerful and designed to be recited every day for thirteen moon cycles.

worrying thoughts and negative self-talk, they are turning their energy downward, to the forgiving, intuitive, judgment-free realm of the heart.

This rising trend to move away from the head and into the heart is a representation of a grand remembering we're undergoing as a species—an understanding that the heart is where the real wisdom lies. Now we're giving you an invitation to go even lower, connecting heart to womb. In an emotionally and spiritually healthy woman, the heart and the womb are teammates, working together in a beautiful, symbiotic relationship. One could not function well without the other, says Marcia Lopez, the founder of Women's True Healing, an organization that supports women at every stage of the pregnancy journey. Marcia brings the wisdom of her Guatemalan heritage into her practice in Southern California, supporting her clients with the ancient arts of Mayan abdominal massage and yoni or vaginal steaming, a practice in which herbal steam is used to cleanse and heal. She's a firm believer in the power of the womb and likens the connection between the womb and the heart to the firm foundation that allows a skyscraper to reach up into the sky. The womb must be open and fortified if the heart is to be big and strong, she says.

If you need motivation to make the effort to connect to your heart and womb—your future baby is it. As Ulrike tells her clients, when you are not afraid to look at the deep stuff that comes up, you actively move toward an awakened or healed womb. This means that your baby won't be imprinted with the old wounds of her mother, father, and what her ancestral line carries.

This kind of clearing is a family affair. Alison Sinatra, a yoga instructor and facilitator of female-centric spiritual retreats (aptly titled "Return of the Queen"), often works closely with women who long to have a child. She encourages these women to take a close look at their own history, reminding them that it's necessary to heal the past to be fully embodied in the present. You can start by bringing attention your birth story.

If possible, ask your mother questions about your conception, her pregnancy, and her labor and delivery experience:

- What was her relationship like with your father when you were conceived?

- Was your conception a surprise?

- Was her pregnancy with you easy or challenging? What about your birth? Why?

- What kind of birth did she have? Vaginal? Breech? C-section? Did she labor for long?

- Did she have any miscarriages, or any other unexpected pregnancy outcomes?

Ask about your grandmother, too. A female baby has all the eggs she will have during her entire life when she is her mother's womb. This means that a piece of you was in your grandmother and that you carry your grandmother's experiences deep within your being as well. Then, when you were in your mother's womb, during your birth, and in the early weeks of your life, you were imprinted with what she experienced. The information you learn about your maternal line can shed important light on your own relationship to pregnancy, birth, and motherhood. If you are able to have this conversation with your mother, know that it could get emotional for her. A lot could come up. Can you hold space for her?

Then it's time to turn your attention to your own history. Paula Mallis, the founder of WMN Space in Los Angeles, also works closely with women who hope to become mothers, leading them in fertility circles and conscious conception workshops. She believes that it is as important to spiritually clean up your system as it is to physically prepare for conception. When left unresolved, the emotional aftershocks that are a result of hard experiences surrounding pregnancy and birth, such as abortions, miscarriages, challenges with previous births, and struggles with fertility, can contribute to blocks that can interfere with conception. Take the time to connect to your womb and feel the energies that are stored there. Then bring your story to the surface, and out of your system, by sharing it with someone you trust.

> The doors to the world of the wild Self are few but precious. If you have a deep scar, that is a door, if you have an old, old story, that is a door. If you love the sky and the water so much you almost cannot bear it, that is a door. If you yearn for a deeper life, a full life, a sane life, that is a door.
>
> —FROM *WOMEN WHO RUN WITH THE WOLVES*, CLARISSA PINKOLA ESTÉS

Becoming familiar with the pregnancy and birth stories of your mother and grandmother, as well as your own, is profoundly healing work. But many experts who work with women hoping to become pregnant also recommend that they pull the lens back beyond the experience of their known relatives. For thousands of years, Ayurvedic lore has taught of *samskaras*, the impressions or grooves that are made on us by our life experiences—both in this lifetime and previous ones—and made especially deep by stress. These imprints express as traits that we can pass down to the next generation, affecting their emotional state, mental outlook, and physical health. Now, new studies in the field of epigenetics is finding that we may carry currents of hurt or trauma that are not our own. Marcia Lopez works with many womb-healing clients who are carrying what she calls intergenerational trauma, ancestral pain that must be cleared if you are to be truly free. She finds that it transcends race—everyone has female ancestors that were oppressed in some way. If you are of Jewish descent, your grandma may have been in the Holocaust; if your family is Cambodian, she may have been part of the genocide; if you're African American, she may have been affected by slavery; if you're Native American, she may have been harmed by colonization—the list goes on and on. For Marcia, ancestral womb clearing is an exceptionally effective process casting out ripples of healing that are generational, communal, and political. She sees it as a catalyst not only for a woman to regain vitality and vivaciousness, as well as the ability to reproduce, but also to give her the opportunity to support the healing we need as humans to move into a better world.

an open relationship with your womb

Thankfully, connecting to your womb is easier than it may seem. It starts by simply placing your hands there. You don't need a yoga mat or a bundle of sage or a Spotify "relax" playlist. All you need are your hands and your intention. You can tune into your womb anytime you have a few quiet moments. This can be while parked in the supermarket parking lot, sitting in a kitchen chair, or in bed when you first wake up or before you fall asleep at night.

Close your eyes, bring your focus down to your hands, and begin to sense into the womb. Notice what you feel or what you see. Remember, this is the feminine dimension—a realm that is often nonlinear and free from boundaries. When you bring consciousness to the womb, you are bringing consciousness to the places that are subconscious and unconscious. The messages you receive may not be clear and easy to decipher at first. This is the dimension of the soul that lives beyond the rational mind. It speaks the subtle language of symbols, images, dreams, intuition, and knowing. But your womb can be straightforward, too, kind of like a no-nonsense best friend that tells it like it is. Marcia Lopez finds the womb to be at once mundane and mystical, ready to communicate messages that are as practical as they are profound. How to hear what it's saying? Just as you can sense how someone riding next to you on the bus is feeling, so can you decipher what your womb wants to share with you, she says. The guidance is often surprisingly simple and direct, along the lines of *stop worrying about what he said, only you know what's right for you,* or *go clean your closet, you'll feel calmer about things when the house is in order.*

Again, connecting with your womb doesn't have to be complex or strange (or any stranger than it already seems). With your hands on your womb, you can simply ask, *Hi, womb, do you have anything to share with me?* And trust the answer, which may come in colors, visions, or feelings. Do you feel a wave of sadness? Or openness? Is the sensation heavy or dark? Or fluttery and agitated? Maybe you don't feel anything at all. Try not to judge the feelings that show up (or don't show up). If you do feel sensations or emotions that are challenging, honor what you are experiencing and allow the energy to come up and out. Ulrike reminds her clients who are doing womb work that the feelings are mostly old things, hard memories from your younger years, childhood, or even from your time in the womb where you felt pain because you were not acknowledged, loved, or received in the way you deserve. The wounding from those experiences is what we perceive when we tune into our womb. And if dialoguing with your womb is too far out there, take a moment to simply thank it for being there for you—as the center of your power and creativity.

> Power connected to love means the womb connected to the heart. When we talk of union, it's about uniting the heart and womb in one energetic center, so we have access to both: love and power.
>
> —MARCIA LOPEZ

forgiveness, the ultimate act of clearing

As you ignite a relationship with your womb and begin to acknowledge hurts that may be stored there, you may find that you're holding on to grudges and resentment that are also taking up valuable spiritual real estate, blocking you from moving into this next chapter of your life. We often closely tend to the emotional injuries that we feel were inflicted by another. We keep them fed and thriving with ongoing accounts of how we were wronged and how the other person is flawed in one or more ways. It may seem as if this holding on is a way of exacting justice for a wrongdoing, an "I'll show them" approach, but you're the only one who suffers in this scenario.

When you forgive others for things that have happened in the past, you create more space in your body, mind, and spirit. Grudges and resentment are like old files on your hard drive. You don't use them anymore, but you are hesitant to let them go, and keeping them makes it impossible for new files to come in; too many can even cause your system to crash. Danica Thornberry, doctor of acupuncture and Oriental medicine, notes that doing emotional reconciliation work like letting go of old wounds and hurts supports the Lung organ system, which in TCM governs the immune system and separating what should stay outside from what belongs inside. Releasing grief and old wounds helps a woman's overall health and immunity and is an essential part of preconception preparation. And there are schools of thought that say that a baby's spirit cannot come into a space that is not open and receptive. You are that space. Think of it as starting a new painting on a clear canvas versus painting on top of an image that is already there. When you take the time, and make the effort, to clear lingering anger, fear, resentment, shame, blame, and guilt, you make room to hold a new creation.

Like any real work that leads to genuine results, forgiving is easier said than done. Until it isn't. Just as you strengthen a muscle in your body by using it regularly, and pushing it past its comfort zone, you can strengthen your forgiveness muscle by doing the same. It looks like this: when you start to feel a current of resentment or anger bubbling up inside you, notice the story you tell yourself:

YOUR OUTER WORLD REFLECTS YOUR INNER WORLD

Not sure how you're feeling? Take a look around you. The state of your space often reflects the state of your mind. Is your home cluttered and unorganized? Dusty and unkempt? Your heart and mind may feel that way, too. You don't need to go full Marie Kondo, but taking the time to attend to your environment can have a tonifying effect on your well-being.

I can't believe he did that to me, he's so selfish, she's so callous, I don't deserve this. Then see if you can drop it. Take inspiration from the pups in your life. Dogs have a built-in nervous system reset. After an outside energy (like a pair of human hands seeking a snuggle) leaves their field, they shake off the residue with a full-body shimmy. You can do the same with a grudge you're holding or a hurt you've experienced. Shake off the sob story before it takes a deeper hold on you. Not forgiving someone takes more energy than forgiving. Stop feeding the resentment beast with your pain. It will starve and you will be free. It's as simple as dropping the need to be right—or to be wronged.

If the cold-turkey approach to forgiveness is a bit out of your reach—not everyone can simply drop it and move on—compassion may be the way out. Remind yourself that nobody is perfect, a list that includes you and the person you're hoping to forgive, and that anyone who has hurt you is likely hurting themselves. And then take it a step further. Regardless of your belief system, you can set a clear intention and then put your desire to change behind it. Some will call this prayer, others a request for help. However you need to frame it, taking the time to state your desire, which can look something like *please help me see this situation in a new light so I can forgive and move on,* can guide you in navigating the bumpy road to true forgiveness. You can write down your request in a journal every day or sit quietly while holding the thought in your mind and heart. There is absolutely no wrong way to ask for help or to make a prayer.

Make a list of the people in your life who you have yet to forgive, both living and deceased, and begin to work your way through each one until you have let go of what you've been holding on to (for inspiration, consider the ultimate act of forgiveness: those individuals who were able to pardon the person who killed a beloved friend or family member). At the top of this list will be your own name. Forgiving yourself is the foundational step to clearing the emotional and spiritual blocks clogging your being. When you reflect on situations in which you hurt someone or moments when you were not acting from your highest self, feel the sting of shame and then let it go. Let it go before your mind gets involved and starts throwing stories your way (they're stories because they're untrue): *I'm messed up. I always do the wrong thing. I'm stupid.* You made mistakes. A lot of them, maybe. Good for you. Mistakes are how you learn. Sometimes the mistakes are small, leaving a minor wake of shame or guilt, and sometimes you

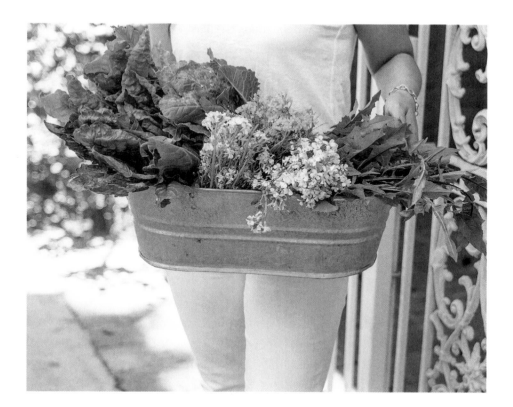

have to blow up your life or the life of another to really absorb the lesson embedded there. Both are okay. For too long now you've been carrying the weight of the hurts you've inflicted on others, and that others have done to you, like a sack of bricks slung over your shoulder. Drop the bundle and notice how light you feel.

review your relationship

The last aspect of clearing that must be attended to is the relationship you have with your partner. As you move closer to the idea of creating a baby together it's essential to ask yourself some key questions, namely:

- Is this the person with whom I want to create a child?

- Are there areas of our relationship that need attention, such as our view on finances or our thoughts on where we want to live or the kind of work we will be doing in the years to come?

- Are there things that I have been hesitant to say but that need to be said?

Now is the time to express thoughts that you have been holding back. This is Clearing, after all! If you're concerned that your partner or spouse may have an unhealthy relationship with alcohol, this is the time to express that feeling. Same goes for his or her relationship to spending, eating, working, or relaxing, for that matter.

This pre-pregnancy preparation phase is also an ideal time to see if you two are aligned in fundamental areas that will influence how you navigate everything from giving birth to the type of education you want your kid(s) to have. If you're all about home birth and Waldorf schooling and he wants a hospital birth and public education, there are some things you'll need to work out. In *The First Forty Days*, we encouraged readers, who we assumed were very pregnant as they read the book, to peel back the layers of their relationship to ensure that they were on the same page as their partners *before* they were thrown into the joyful chaos of caring for an infant. Just months away from

HO'OPONOPONO: A HAWAIIAN PRACTICE OF FORGIVENESS

Translated literally, the Hawaiian word "Ho'oponopono" means to put in order, correct, rectify, make orderly or neat. In other words, to clear what's weighing you down. The practice is integrated into teachings led by priests, shamans, and Buddhists and used by therapists to help you return to right relation with yourself and those in your life.

To practice, repeat these four phrases for a minute in the morning and at night, working up to five minutes each session. Bring your attention to someone you'd like to forgive, someone you may have hurt, or focus on forgiving yourself. If you practice regularly, the results can be extraordinary.

I am sorry / Please forgive me / Thank you / I love you

birth, there was no time to waste in exploring hot-button issues surrounding child care and finances. In this pre-pregnancy preparation phase the urgency is not as pressing, but we still implore you to have these very real discussions with your partner as soon as you can. Many (okay, most) of these topics are quite deep and personal and it may take time to find resolution if you disagree. Starting early will give you time to seek outside help if necessary. Your relationship with your partner will be your baby's first experience of what it means to relate to another human being—it's worth the investment.

readiness is a two-way street

As you turn your sights to becoming a mother, your desire to procreate can pick up speed and velocity and before you know it you've left important factors languishing in its dust. You may find that you want to skip ahead before you've regulated your cycle, wrangled your stress levels, or shifted away from harmful habits. You may also blaze past the other human being who matters in this equation. It's very easy to use the perceived restraints of your biological clock as an excuse to steamroll over your partner's thoughts and feelings about parenthood, but it's important to confirm that you're both ready in the same way at the same time. If you feel ready to become a parent but your partner says he's not yet there, it's important to respect his point of view. There's a common belief, usually tossed about irreverently with your girlfriends or older female relatives, that men are never ready and it's a woman's job to push them into parenthood or the species won't proliferate. That line of thinking completely discounts the experience, and intuitive foresight, of men.

If you think he'll come around once he's holding his irresistibly adorable baby, you're glossing over a deeper issue that can calcify into resentment that may be very difficult to dissolve as the relationship progresses. Even though he's not the one who will be pregnant or giving birth, your partner's life will be forever altered by the arrival of a baby. He will likely have to adjust the way he works, and how he moves through the world, maybe even putting a dream or goal on the back burner. Take the time in the early months of preparation, before you even start moving toward conception, to really listen to each other's needs. Don't sidestep this preliminary work. Your life together will be so much more harmonious if you embark on parenthood from a place of agreement and love. Find the courage to take in the full spectrum of his experience even if it feels scary or uncertain. If you are not in agreement, understand that it may not resolve overnight. Prepare to have a series of challenging conversations and work toward creating a contract that outlines what parenthood will look like for both of you—for example, you may agree that you will dive into his savings to subsidize childcare, while your hard-won new business funds will remain untouched. While it may seem formal to get your agreement down on paper, it

To have a conversation with your uterus and to live a womb-centered life. It's not scary—it's cool!

—MARCIA LOPEZ

can give you both a roadmap to follow—something that can be especially useful when you're drowning in the sea of depletion and overwhelm that can grip brand-new parents.

At the heart of all of this is the broader realization that the becoming you're headed toward is about more than becoming a mother; it's about becoming a family—and doing so from a place of peace and accord.

When you take the time to sit with and practice the Clearing ideas and techniques in this chapter, you are giving a gift to yourself, your partner, and your future child. As you dive in, keep in mind that just like every other practice or new way of thinking held in these pages, Clearing is an unfolding; it's a process of discovery that doesn't happen overnight. It's not a quick erase of the chalkboard or a quick run to the dump. For some it can take a few weeks, for others a few years, yet with steady and courageous determination to heal and become free, Clearing is a gradual but defined way to step into the light.

SIT IN SILENCE
WITH YOUR PARTNER

As a key aspect of his detailed conception ceremony (see Conceiving, page 147, for more on the practice), Dr. Jay Lokhande has couples practice this silent breathing exercise together. Communication with language is essential, of course, but sometimes simply sitting together tenderly and quietly is the fastest way back to each other.

Sit across from each other, either cross-legged on the bed or floor or in chairs, with knees touching. Gently synchronize your breathing. Breathe together for two to ten minutes. Then sit back-to-back so you can feel each other breathing. Breathe like that for about fifteen minutes. Consciously breathing with your partner like this every day will bring you into harmony with each other, making you aligned and prepared to create strong progeny.

fortifying

I stand at the large gas-fired stove that is the heart of my kitchen, stirring a pot of bone broth before a few women on their pre-pregnancy path, my growing teen daughters joining our circle for the afternoon. In the kitchen, I feel I can claim the title Wise One. They say it takes ten thousand hours to master a subject—when it comes to feeding women, I'm surely on my way by now! As I take in the spread of ingredients I plan to use today—cleansing burdock root, immune-building enoki mushrooms, Kidney-building wild salmon and walnuts—I smile at them like they are old friends, hoping the other women catch this spirit.

When you make great ingredients your staples, and commit to using them often, you'll find those nutritional needs tend to be met.

W e're gathering in a "preconception kitchen" today to learn some new recipes, though in truth, it could equally be called a "pregnancy kitchen," a "postpartum kitchen," or simply a "woman's kitchen," for the tenets and the dishes that support a woman at every stage of her reproductive life are similar; it's just that certain ingredients move more into the foreground at some times versus others. This is *my* most personal contribution to awakening fertility within each woman; I'm a passionate advocate for homemade, hearty food, and I strive to wake up the part of her that cooks!

Preparing our meal in this earthy, easy fashion, I can almost feel my aunties approving. To help "get the baby room ready," as they would say, we keep it simple—no fancy food, no fancy trouble. Fortifying is the complement to Preparing's clearing of the field; by getting our hands on humble and wholesome ingredients from Mother Nature, we start to build up the soil of our inner ecosystem and enrich the body with nutrients—our version of luscious mulch, glorious compost, and the finest soil amendments!—to become as rich and fertile as it can be. Yet it's more than just bodily nourishment that's occurring in this preconception kitchen as we chop and stir, wooden spoons at the ready. We are fortifying our *relationship* with food, developing a stronger connection with cooking and repairing frayed bonds if they exist. Kitchen time is a moment to slow down, to remember you have a body and it wants you to listen to it. Laughing, I encourage each woman to put her hands on her midsection. "Go on," I say. "Ask your ovaries, your uterus, 'What do you want to eat today?'" I'm convinced that each one of us knows more about what we need than we think we do.

I believe that strengthening your relationship with food is more important during the prelude to pregnancy than at any other phase in your life, save, perhaps, for the forty weeks of gestation itself. It starts with a choice: *I choose to feed myself well!* Just like getting clear on your romantic relationship is paramount when turning toward parenting—*Yes, I want to create a family with you*—I encourage each woman to bring equal conviction to her body. Fortifying starts with an intent to support yourself physically and build your reserves, for the passage ahead will demand a lot from you and feeding yourself properly can't be an afterthought on a busy day or something you kinda-sorta intend to do (but kinda-sorta forget, more often than not). The good news is that once you make this inner declaration, you'll find it's reciprocal; devote a part of yourself to health-giving food and it in turn will deliver incredible support to you. Cooking vibrant and enriching food not only helps conserve your fertility potential and builds your reserves; the act of getting your hands a little dirty in the kitchen helps you sink your roots deeper into your life so that you can bloom.

Because here's the obvious but sometimes little-discussed reality of making a baby: every aspect of reproduction requires an abundance of energy and high-grade raw materials, and they're derived from food. The monthly creation and orchestration of hormones like estrogen and progesterone depend on well-digested, healthy natural fats, amino acids from proteins, as well as vitamins and minerals. For these sex hormones to stay at proper levels and ratios, a steady stream of fiber-filled and detoxifying plant foods are required to help the liver do its essential clearing and synthesizing work. The plush lining of a welcoming baby room (the uterus) flourishes when blood is "strong," as

Building reserves in advance pays back infinitely. The minute a mom gets undernourished, her child will start feeling that their mom isn't full and isn't getting her needs met, and then the child becomes a hot mess! If we can avoid that depletion, the baby so often falls into alignment.

—JAPA KHALSA

traditionalists say—fortified with iron and other minerals—made by a Spleen system working at its best. (It also helps to ensure correct levels of warming progesterone.) Meanwhile, the egg and sperm need the amino acids from well-absorbed proteins as well as many micronutrients; the membranes of each cycle's maturing egg get positively bouncy when nature's best fats are well absorbed, while the sperm flourish if a symphony of selenium, B_{12}, folate, and zinc have helped get them in tip-top shape to earn their chance at "catching the egg." And once a fertilized egg settles into the baby room, it's game on as the act of transforming into a baby gets under way in a phenomenon of extraordinary growth and development, and the way it happens impacts a child's life over the long term! None of this happens by magic or sheer intention; it takes continuous material input, actual building blocks delivered via the food that you choose to eat. (So do the phases after pregnancy—breastfeeding and mom's postpartum recovery are powerfully impacted by how well your nutritional reserves are filled before, during, and after birth, as we describe in *The First Forty Days*.)

> Become too heady about it, and the act of eating can start to be stripped of its heart and soul. And what kind of start to mothering would that be?

The nutritional requirements for even getting *up* to the starting line of pregnancy are nothing to sneeze at. Yet while it's important to take them seriously, after cooking for and with women over the years, I'm passionate that the responsibility shouldn't feel weighty. Building yourself up before pregnancy shouldn't be a relentless, single-minded project like a quarterback working overtime to bulk up and make the team. It shouldn't give you anxiety that you aren't doing it "right." Sages in my family's tradition teach that fear weakens the Kidney organ system—the very aspect we want to strengthen for procreation! Furthermore, fretting hurts the Spleen, and without our dear Spleen calmly and reliably digesting our food, we're up the creek without a paddle. So a big breath and a serving of balance is in order.

As you explore the fourth realm of preconception care, Fortifying, consider that eating is a multidimensional act: it's about the physical nutrients you absorb and assimilate into your blood and tissues, and it's about the invisible vitality or *chi* they hold that feeds *your chi*, your personal vitality. The benefits of eating well include the ways essential fatty acids support brain health, for example, and *also* the ways that sweet, salty, or bitter tastes stimulate corresponding organ systems to function their best, which in turn affects your outlook and mood. Ask anyone well versed in acupuncture, Ayurveda, or energy medicine, and they'll even tell you that the vitality of food is influenced by your intention as you prepare it. I love the personal, intimate aspect of eating the most. Food is as much about memory, and dreams, and desires as it is about ratios of protein to carbohydrate. It's the most visceral way we experience the effects of changing seasons: the way a cooling summer cucumber or grounding autumn squash feels when you eat it can remind you that, as TCM teaches, you are a microcosm of the macrocosm, influenced by the rhythms of nature. Food can be a thread that ties you to your long-distant past, if you discover that the diet that works best for you is shaped by the foods your ancestors ate and the lands they came from. With practice, your meals can even help you connect with your inner medicine woman, a medium for hearing your body's quiet messages.

All this to say, while getting enriching ingredients into your body (and your partner's) is deeply empowering, become too heady about it—*I must eat a can of sardines daily, I must, I must!*—and the act of eating can start to be stripped of its heart and soul. And what kind of start to mothering would that be?

Remember the traditional credo that says for a woman to bear fruit she must be "gently nourished"? I translate that to mean, consistently fed ingredients that deliver essential support to her organ systems, accruing in goodness over time and helping to create ongoing conditions of balance and harmony, but with no forcing and no anxiety allowed. The best way to approach this is to start early! Begin to eat as if you were pregnant months or years before you seek to conceive, cleaning out the foods that deplete or tax your system and filling your plate with foods that help, heal, and strengthen. So many women are starting out depleted today, struggling with some combination of adrenal

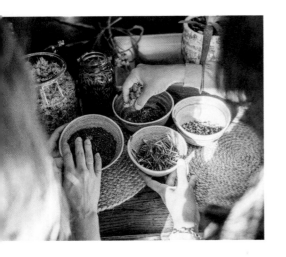

fatigue, excessive stress, weak digestion, or the depletions of key nutrients such as B vitamins, including folate; vitamins C and E; selenium and magnesium; and the antioxidant CoQ10, as well as imbalances in protective gut flora, that can happen after years of taking hormonal birth control. Or simply years of shirking a nutritious daily diet. On top of that, so much of our food is grown or processed in ways that strip it of nutrition, and then cocktails of contaminants from the air, water, and soil get layered in, too. We face a few challenges our predecessors did not. Fortify yourself ahead of the game and you get plenty of time to address depletions, discover the foods that serve your body best, and kick bad habits to the curb. You can even accommodate going rogue here and there without it taking too much of a toll—a laughter-filled pizza night with friends or cocktails on date night, in my opinion, is part of a healthy diet if it contributes to your happiness and sense of connection. I always tell my clients that eating better happens in forward spurts, then small backward slides, then another few steps forward—you make progress over time, and it's all good. I've found 90 percent clean and healthy and 10 percent fun food works well for most.

Crucially, starting early lets you gradually transition into a healthy prenatal diet. You don't have to pivot at the last minute—*I'm pregnant! What do I eat now?*—or make an awkward U-turn. I've always thought it takes two years for a couple to know they truly want to parent together; taking two years to truly get in the groove with good eating makes equal sense to me!

If starting early isn't an option—maybe you're set on making a baby just a few short months from now—the approach shifts a few degrees: you'll want to be more intentional about consuming nourishing and fortifying foods and less tolerant of sugary, junk-foody, or boozy messing around. (And if you have any known or suspected food sensitivities, you'll want to be a real

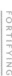

Goody-Two-shoes!) Know that the foods you and your partner eat today will greatly influence the health of the sperm that is presently forming and that might meet its destined egg in three months, which is really the bare minimum of time to dial up your diet for optimal benefits. That egg is presently starting its important three-month maturation or ripening phase in the follicle, too. Meanwhile you'll want to be working hard at building the reserves a growing baby will require: Experts say it takes about three months to build great reserves of folate, a B vitamin most of us know is pivotal for early fetal development, and our wise ones who practice Chinese medicine say that in three months of eating to serve weak or depleted organs, significant cycle rebalancing often occurs. Every bite counts! Yet even so the question remains, can you make this fast-track project easeful and enjoyable—something that helps you bloom rather than bogs you down? Whether you're on the slow continuum like I was, building up my relationship and intuition around eating through my twenties, or whether you're taking the fast track, know that it's really worth putting food first. You're setting yourself up well for pregnancy and will soon have a sound eating style nicely established.

the third way

In my kitchen, preconception nourishment starts with a deep respect for food. After all, a vital, balanced diet is your ticket to helping preserve your treasure chest of jing, the legacy of health and longevity you're planning to pass on to your offspring! So I always begin with the question, "What wisdom can I take from the old ways?" My people (and yours, too, wherever they're from) were eating "real food" long before the phrase was coined—this foodie term simply means eating unprocessed whole foods sourced in old-school ways that ensure they retain their full nutritional power. Our great-grandmothers and grandfathers had free-roaming chickens in their backyard and cooked nose-to-tail style, never wasting a scrap of any meat or fish sourced; they used an abundance of local, seasonal produce, beans, and legumes; prepared grains in methodical ways to make them digestible; and fermented foods to make them last. The old folks in the community would cluck and smile over babies with chubby cheeks, big smiles, and mischievous curiosity, saying those were the result of the good foods they'd created for the family. (When I discovered the traditional preconception and pregnancy findings of Weston A. Price I recognized the themes immediately—cultures and tribes from every part of the globe were doing Chinese granny cooking!)

A garden that's been carefully enriched, its soil built up over time, is a world away from a plot that's been left unattended or half-forgotten. When you do this for yourself, my how your garden grows!

However, I like to interpret the guidance from the past through a present-time filter, always asking, *What looks good today at the market when I shop, and moreover, what are women telling me they want to eat today?* Like my forbearers, my approach is omnivorous, with gratitude for every type of food nature offers us. But I also acknowledge that we are all individual; not every body responds the same way to every food, and there are layers of thought and emotion around eating that are personal to each person. There are also trends, interests, and seasons to factor in—all kinds of things inspire our appetite! I'm not a doctor handing over a food prescription—I'd never want to tell you that you have to eat one food or another. My way is more artistic and intuitive; I want you to imagine your body as a wondrous ecosystem that will do its very best to give you what you long for, if you lovingly tend to its needs.

This perspective is a little different from a technical prenatal diet book. It's looser—after all, you're not in the prenatal stage yet, not yet in the purview of midwives and OB-GYNs checking your blood levels and handing you rigorous nutrition guides. And it echoes what I was steeped in growing up; where the Western approach to nutrition itemizes macro- and micronutrients, with recommended daily allowances stamped on foods in bold font, and vitamins or minerals linked to specific functions, the Chinese understanding assesses the energetic qualities of foods in addition to their physical components—asking, are they warming or cooling, stimulating or calming, and evaluating their effect on your overall balance. Traditional Chinese medicine tends to talk of how foods help create a harmonious inner environment in which blood circulates smoothly and chi or vitality flows or resonates fully—two things particularly important to arrive at the state in which "blood and chi are overflowing," as Danica Thornberry teaches—and says that the way into this is by nourishing the organ systems as well as removing blocks in the meridians. Though the philosophy might sound esoteric, the outcomes are very tangible: glowing skin, shiny hair, youthful resiliency—and when it comes to reproduction, those cheery, chubby-cheeked babies!

This is why I ask women to place their hands on their abdomen and, even if it feels utterly weird, to try to feel into what their body might be saying. It's about getting out of your head with food and connecting to your body. When I cook for myself or for other women, I'm always envisioning these interconnected systems, honoring them, thanking them for giving us life and health, and asking if I can help them if they're weak.

In my ideal world, a woman's mate would do the same thing—he'd put his hands on his lower body and feel into his reproductive system for what it needs to thrive. A pipe dream, I know! But in the Chinese tradition, men are super-conscious of how food affects their virility—to a fault, consuming some pretty strange (or environmentally unethical) things like donkey meat, silkworms, and liquor infused with tiger bone to build up vigor and heat in the body, sometimes spending oodles of money on *nanke*, or men's medicine, to get that "raging bull" feeling going on. They've made the connection: robust sperm and subsequent healthy offspring are the product of supercharged nutrition.

The story of women and food can often be a story of extremes—maybe you're familiar with it in your own life. Too much food or not enough; being rigid and unyielding around eating or falling into inertia or rote patterns; overly preoccupied with what's on your plate or mindlessly munching on foods empty of real nutrition. It can even create a kind of interpersonal disharmony, where you can feel so passionate about your way, you inadvertently critique others for *theirs*. Add in pregnancy, which raises the stakes higher (and seems to make every self-care subject a hot button issue), and instead of being joyous, preconception eating can start to feel dogmatic or even stifling!

Fortifying yourself before pregnancy does not, in my opinion, have to mean chowing on nutrient-dense animal foods and their derivatives for breakfast, lunch, dinner, and snacks daily (though I believe these foods in moderation and frequent rotation are important for pre-pregnancy fortifying). Nor do I personally choose to zero in on isolated nutrients that must be acquired in measured amounts daily, checked off a to-do list. In nature, nutrients don't exist in isolation; they come combined together as a whole food! I find my way to the stove by imagining what the organ systems need to get to that abundant, brimming state of strong blood, vital chi, and balanced and harmonious organs: the Kidney needs building foods, the Liver needs clarifying foods, the Spleen needs digestible, soothing foods—and then I color this with a generally warming approach, which tends to support most women best. I put less of my attention on what *not* to eat, because frankly I think most women already know the broad strokes here. It's not news: sugar, highly processed foods and junk foods, excesses of refined carbohydrates, processed vegetable oils, and fried foods are all inflammatory in nature, and the raging fires of inflammation do not create the environment for the easeful flow and dance of hormonal and reproductive health!

I prefer to focus on the positives: *What foods can I choose that will help, heal, and happify?* (Yes, that's a word, I checked the dictionary.) The challenge for most women is consistently preparing and cooking good-for-us foods, and getting to the place where it's second nature to fill every plate or bowl with goodness, without too much thought or struggle. That's why I preach a hybrid

> When you take a basic ancestral approach, you find a consistency among very diverse peoples and diets. The most important sacred foods used during pregnancy were consistently the foods that were highest in animal-source fats and fat-soluble nutrients.
>
> —NORA GEDGAUDAS,
> author, clinician, and ancestral nutrition expert

style: honoring older wisdom about sacred, fortifying foods *and* honoring your own body wisdom, learning to listen in to how foods feel to you and noticing their energetic effects. Honoring yourself also means acknowledging that you are by nature in ebb and flow—you need different kinds of nutritional support to address different moments, like the phases of your cycle, shifts in your stress level, and changes in climate and season. Acknowledging old wisdom and present-time fluctuations helps you arrive at a peaceful center, a third way that's neither overly perfectionist about eating nor passive and checked out, and that is engaged, curious, and intuitive. It's a great place to be, for it will serve you well when you're charged with feeding another being, or an entire family, all looking at you like chicks in the nest, hungry beaks open! You'll feel confident about choosing and preparing the ingredients that will keep your loved ones well fed.

honest accounting

Chances are you have tried various eating styles and experimented with what works for you. Maybe your pantry is well stocked with whole foods, you're picky about where you eat out, or at least feel savvy about the pitfalls of foods filled with additives. Yet even with this level awareness, if you're like many women the first question to address is the simplest: Do I really *feed* myself? Do I eat enough, and do I give myself the permission to slow down—to pause, breathe, and eat, with no distractions and no racing through it—so my digestive system can get the most out of my meals?

No matter where you're starting from, Fortifying starts with taking a full accounting of yourself, as wise one Tibby Plasse told us. She's a mother and biodynamic farming advocate in Idaho's Teton Valley (and an Eastern Idaho chapter head for the Weston A. Price Foundation, a touchstone of the real food movement). An honest accounting includes assessing your current relationship to food, asking whether you consistently eat nourishing meals at the same times each day or are all over the map, and if you make regular time to shop and prepare food or dodge meals with caffeine or snacks because you don't.

(Turn to page 207, by the way, to find snack recipes that bridge the gap between meals healthfully.) It involves looking at how you eat in relation to others: Do you and your mate—potential parents-to-be and joint heads-of-family—prepare and eat food together most days, and by the way, is there some joy or bonding around feeding each other?

If you already have children, have you fallen into the habit of feeding child first, mom last (like picking at his leftovers instead of making a meal)? Tibby says this accounting might include a regional twist, like asking if your diet is hearty enough to fuel you in cold climes or if you're hewing to a diet better suited to the tropics. It might include actual fiscal accounting, like whether you can shift some of your food budget from eating out to grocery spending for home cooking, and find a little extra to spend on high-quality ingredients. And Tibby says it should include a literal accounting of your plate. Do they comprise a balance of fresh vegetables, moderate portions of protein (whether animal- or plant-based), and good fats (think saturated, monosaturated, and omega-3s) to keep you satiated, help you absorb vitamins and minerals, and keep your blood sugar stable? (Constant spikes and drops in blood sugar disrupt your insulin, which can over time negatively affect your sex hormones.)

Fortifying means first and foremost shoring up any weak spots in this pivotal relationship. Making changes to your diet and committing to cooking more may be easier said than done—it can involve finding entirely new food sources and reorganizing your schedule and social life!—but what if you felt into the lifelong responsibility you will have for your child and turned that force of will to yourself? (Force of will, by the way, is regulated by the Kidneys, another reason to build them up!) Rest assured that changes are not *necessarily* challenges. They're opportunities to invest in your health and that of your future family, and if you're willing to make that investment, you'll get off to a much stronger start than if you aren't. Should resistance to carving more time in the kitchen come up, try reframing cooking from drudge-filled chore to a daily chance for connection: to your body and your intuition, to your home and your partner, and even to nature and the greater cosmos, as you tune into the rhythms of seasonal and local harvest.

As you explore the realm of Fortifying, my hope is you will lean on the recipes in this book to discover new ways to feed yourself and your partner well. They're inspired by five aspects of your body according to TCM that, when well tended, will help you gradually arrive at the overflowing state in which you are primed and ready for baby making. Consider them like five threads of a balanced and harmonious preconception tapestry. They're not intended to comprise a formula or a program, per se, but just a way to orient yourself as you put together a daily plate or bowl. Besides, there's no one-size-fits-all when it comes to eating. Each person will find a way that suits their constitution best. Let these universal tenets inspire you as you consider what to eat.

Looking at food in this way doesn't mean you're ignoring the pragmatic minutiae of the nutrients a woman moving toward conception (and later, her growing baby) will want to have at the ready. It's just looking from a different angle; what we find is that the foods that serve each of the five aspects are chock-full of nourishing fats and building proteins and strengthening iron and brain-boosting DHA and cleansing phytonutrients from plants and much, much more. The old ways knew what they were doing! When you make great ingredients your staples, and commit to using them often, you'll find those nutritional needs tend to be met. And my hope is that you will make these foods with your mate; his body will be equally served by all that follows, and his responsibility to put fresh, high-energy foods in place of poor ones is equal to yours!

1. PRESERVE YOUR JING

To best conserve the treasure chest or inheritance of health that is at the root of your fertility potential, the old ways advocate a balanced diet of natural foods, cooked in simple, loving ways, and consumed at regular, consistent intervals and in a state of gratefulness and calm. Avoiding substances that deplete jing, like excessive caffeine, is wise (the herbalist Chad Cornell always balances coffee with a jing tonic, his favorites being the adaptogenic herbs ashwaghanda

FOUR SIMPLE ACCOUNTING QUESTIONS

- Am I willing to make time for cooking or sourcing quality food?

- When I don't feed myself well, what tends to be the obstacle, and how can I avoid that?

- What are my strengths when it comes to feeding my body, and what are my weaknesses (not enough vegetables, reliance on processed foods, leaving too much time between meals, etc.).

- Is my partner on board with eating this way?

and schizandra). Removing irritants and aggravants like foods that you suspect or know trigger inflammatory immune system responses in your body, will also, in my opinion, help preserve jing. (Gluten, dairy, eggs, and corn tend to be the most common.)

From an Ayurvedic perspective, this holistic and conscious approach to eating contributes to the body's production of ojas, which is a thirty-day process that starts with digesting food; as you recall, both jing and ojas are considered to be the subtle essence from which sperm and egg are made. As the Ayurvedic wise one Dr. Jay Lokhande told us, "This is about your whole *life,* not just a diet! There is no absolute single science which can capture it." The discipline around eating, the thoughts you think, and the emotions you feel while you eat all contribute to the *smoothness* of living that helps balance and harmony express. It can be good to think of jing as a *potential*—an essence that will imbue life force into you and your offspring. It's subtle, so it requires equally subtle care. Finding that third way, neither too much nor too little of any food group on a plate, and not getting overly rigid but celebrating contrast in seasonal variety, color, and texture—physically embodying the balance of yin and yang on the plate!—are also part of the daily way you do your *Jing* Thing.

In the prelude to pregnancy, you want to lend your inherited jing some earthly ("post-heaven") support. Tending to the trio of yin organs—the Kidney, Liver, and Spleen—is paramount here. The Kidney organ system is the epicenter of reproductive energy and also your source of courage, willpower, and "I can do this!" energy. They're your foundation of life—but hard-and-fast living tires them out. When you nourish your Kidneys, you shore up depletion, take in the proteins and fats required for healthy hormone function and regular menstrual cycles, and build up the reserves that a baby will need for growth. Many of the foods that nourish the Kidneys also build up the blood, which is critical before pregnancy, because what will deliver oxygen and nutrients to a baby? Your strong, well-circulating blood. You also want to build up blood throughout your cycle, to balance the blood you lose each time you menstruate and help the uterus build its new lining.

Our wise ones unanimously pointed to small, regular portions of super nutrient-rich foods such as bone broths, marrow, and organ meats and beef, lamb, bison, and wild game, all ideally slow cooked, better yet cooked on the bone, as the densest source of Kidney support. So are pasture-raised eggs, especially the yolks, and seafood—think clams, oysters, fatty (and mercury-safer) fish like sardines, mackerel, wild salmon, and eel, for men in particular—just picture the affinity between eel and sperm and yes, eel and penis!—and even the crème de la crème of jing-supportive fish foods: the tiny eggs known as roe (or if you're feeling spendy, caviar). Full-fat dairy foods like grass-fed butter and ghee and yogurt and kefir, ideally in their raw form, can also be deeply Kidney-nourishing (if dairy works for your body; ghee is lactose free and a terrific, nurturing fat for all).

These traditional foods, ideally sourced grass fed, pasture raised, or wild caught, have an almost medicinal effect when it comes to preconception. They help fill your reserve tank from low to brimming. They combine protein and saturated fats together, which help rebuild any hormone deficiencies and pad the adrenals, helping to restore what is lost each day to cumulative stress; from a Western point of view, we know that this repertoire of powerhouse foods contain the most potent levels or forms of fat-soluble vitamins A, D, and K available, as well as B vitamins, especially B_6 and B_{12}, choline, iron, and zinc, and

FORTIFYING

the essential omega-3 acids like DHA that help baby's brain develop and keep mom's mood stable after birth.

But it's not just animal foods that do this. Your Kidneys gain strength from all kinds of mineral-rich foods and the plant world has plenty to offer: nuts and seeds like black sesame, walnut, and chia are especially good, as are dark-colored plant foods like kidney beans, black and adzuki beans, dark leafy greens, and seaweed and algae, full of trace minerals like iodine to support the thyroid (iodine works synergistically with selenium, which is rich in Brazil nuts, mushrooms, and oysters among other foods.) Bee pollen and royal jelly support Kidneys too. TCM says the Kidneys are governed by the water element and resonate with the taste of salt. Thus, savory soups, with mineral-rich ingredients, spiked with sea salt, are your friends in this department! While many of these mineral-rich foods not surprisingly also build the blood (especially liver, with its sky-high levels of B_{12} and iron, and to a lesser but still meaningful effect, seaweeds and micro algae like spirulina and chlorella!), so do dark chicken, grass-fed gelatin, and dark berries including goji berries, beets, and dates. In Chinese medicine, it's not uncommon to use herbs like dong quai to build the blood, too.

If your diet is currently wholly plant-based, and/or if you are concerned about the sustainability of eating animal products, as many of us are, this might create a conundrum. Each of the wise ones we consulted, experts who've tended to modern women at all stages of the maternal journey, gently suggested a reframing in this case: ask yourself, Would I be open to gratefully receiving some animal-sourced product, even if only for this procreation-centered phase of my life? Japa Khalsa says, "We honor ahimsa, the practice of non-violence, but we also do not want to harm your own body by depriving it of what it needs." Bone broth can be a way into this, sipped alone or used in warming soups; perhaps you'd consider consuming small portions of organ meats as the traditionalists suggested, with reverence. Both these foods let you get a lot of nutrition affordably from sustainably and ethically raised animals. At the very least, would orange-yolked eggs, seafood, shellfish, cod liver oil, and lashings of grass-fed butter make the cut? Japa also reiterates that "Mom knows best. Follow your inner guidance and knowing." Should you choose to avoid

Wise one Lauren Curtain taught us how eating liver and kidney, pastured beef, chicken, and eggs, fatty fish, oysters, and broccoli ensure you get CoQ10, an antioxidant that fuels your mitochondria to make energy. This is key for egg health, especially as you get older and lose some of your natural cellular energy while being exposed to more inflammatory toxins. Your eggs are profuse with mitochondria and they need high-level support to help their chromosomes line up as they should and accomplish the feats of fertilization, implantation and growth. Another good reason to consume those Kidney-building foods! It's incredible how traditional knowledge and modern science align.

all animal or seafood products, it's important to acknowledge that in some key areas, such as the long-chain fatty acid DHA, vitamins A, B_{12}, and K_2, and choline, your diet may leave you and your future offspring lacking; the guidance of a practitioner very well versed in nutrition could serve your family well.

3. SUPPORT THE SPLEEN AND WARM THE BODY

In Chapter 3, you read about the foods the Liver needs to help keep your body in balance—things like a steady supply of vegetables, including bitter greens, cruciferous ones, and beets, soothing extra-virgin olive oil, and turmeric. It's equally vital to keep the Spleen's requirements top of mind—sometimes referred to as the Spleen/Stomach, it's like the pot on the stove of digestion where food is broken down and absorbed so it can nourish all your organs and tissues, and build up your blood and *chi*. If you want to get to "overbrimming," a contented Spleen, working side by side with a happy, clear Liver, is where it's at. (In TCM, the Spleen makes the blood; the Liver helps it proliferate or circulate.)

The Spleen resonates with the taste of sweet. This doesn't mean dessert! Think sweet-tasting root vegetables like yams, pumpkin, and squash (topped

A NOTE ON PROTEIN

Start including protein at every meal now to support your hormonal health (and ensure you feel sated) and you'll get in the habit of including moderate portions at every meal. This means during pregnancy and after (when protein needs are high!) you'll be well set, and might even dial it up. Animal-derived proteins are not hard to figure out, but remember there are lots of plant-sourced ones, too, such as lentils, mung beans, brown rice, kidney, lima, pinto, and black beans, quinoa, other whole grains, and hemp and sunflower seeds. (But skip the unfermented soy products such as soy milk, tofu, and soy-based energy bars and desserts. Unfermented soy is estrogen-disrupting.)

with nourishing fats like grass-fed butter, ghee, extra-virgin olive oil, avocado oil, or unrefined sesame oil or coconut oil). Include lots of warm-cooked greens and colorful vegetables, steamed, braised, and cooked into stews, drizzled with fats to ensure their vitamins and minerals are easily absorbed. The Spleen is also nurtured by well-cooked whole grains—assuming grains digest well for you—ideally soaked and sprouted first to reduce the naturally occurring anti-nutrients that inhibit vitamin and mineral absorption. (Use organic grains whenever you can to avoid fertility-harming herbicides and pesticides.) Grass-fed beef is considered a tonic for a weak Spleen, which if not gently corrected can express as anemia.

Warm, soupy, and congee-type foods are heaven to the Spleen, especially in colder months when body heat is precious. They require less energy to digest, which helps the body maintain its warmth. If you're familiar with *The First Forty Days*, you know that I consider inner warmth to be a woman's ally in preconception, pregnancy, and postpartum phases, especially in our era of Kidney and adrenal fatigue. (TCM considers a Kidney yang deficiency to be a precursor to a "cold" uterus, which is not conducive to healthy cycles or successful implantation. The baby room needs to be cozy!) Add some warm-propertied garlic and onion to these soups, and warming meat, too, and you've got a winning combo.

In contrast, salads and raw foods, so often seen as a cornerstone of good eating, are not always the Spleen's friend, especially in colder months. They are energetically cold, and this cold can potentially penetrate the energy channels that support the reproductive system. Unless it's high summer, enjoying raw produce in smaller amounts and noticing your own tendencies to feel gently warmed or, as can sometimes happen, totally chilled by what you eat is a wise idea. Rest assured there are lots of ways to preserve your body's inner warmth. A morning chai tea with warming spices like cinnamon and ginger, frequent sips of hot water throughout the day (a time-tested trick for supporting digestion and circulation), and a moratorium on iced drinks and freezing foods, unless you're out sweating on the tennis court in mid-July! The warming quality is not the same as the mouth-burning heat from super-spicy ingredients. Moderate, steady warmth that does not spike to overheated is ideal for both the woman and for the man because sperm thrives in the middle way, neither too hot nor too chilled.

Nurturing the Spleen also means taking care not to let too much sugar overwhelm the spleen. This can contribute to disharmonies like PCOS and other metabolic dysfunction and set a risky precedent for pregnancy. Keep an eye on total carbohydrate intake, prioritizing high-fiber foods like vegetables, beans, and legumes over refined carbs (especially the white ones) and find your own personal sweet spot—everyone's body tolerates carbohydrates differently. The common denominator? Get sugars as low as they'll go—in the Recipes section (page 164) you'll find some low-sugar ways to enjoy sweet flavors. Another motivation to take good care of these organs? When the Spleen and Kidney are in balance, your skin and beauty get a radiant glow!

4. EAT FOR CHI

Chi is a little different from the human health inheritance known as jing. You could say it's even more subtle—it is the vibration of life in all of nature and all the cosmos. It's the vitality that brings life to cells, tissues, and organs. Chi is like the voltage of your cellular batteries ensuring your whole system lights up—you want it to be nice and high.

The wise ones say that the foods that hold the highest chi or vitality are fresh vegetables and fruits, and you and your mate want to enjoy lots of them, not only because their high fiber helps to move used-up hormones and broken-down toxins out through your GI tract, and they keep your Liver peppy, but because their rainbow of colors offers myriad compounds to support optimal fertility and preconception health. As the excellent TCM fertility book *Making Babies* describes, the greens in kale, chard, collards, and seaweed, among others, fill you with folate, iron, B vitamins, and more; reds from peppers and tomatoes deliver sperm count–boosting lycopene, blues and purples of eggplant, red cabbage, and dark berries offer toxin-busting antioxidant support, and white allium vegetables (garlic, onion, and chives) contribute important antibacterial and antifungal properties to protect you against fertility-blocking infections. Bromelain, the enzyme in pineapple, by the way, is purported to support implantation if eaten in the two-day ovulatory window, though rock-solid confirmation of this is hard to find.

According to wise one Dr. Linda Lancaster, who's spent four decades of dowsing (reading the energy field) of food for her patients, there's a very significant difference between the vitality of organic produce, especially local and seasonal ones recently picked, and conventional produce grown with chemicals and often grown and picked many thousands of miles away. Whenever possible, choose the former. The most vital vegetables of all? Those might just be sprouts, bursting with the energy of new life! This type of raw food is fine to use in smaller amounts as a final touch to your bowl and plate; nutritionally, sprouts and microgreens like broccoli, arugula, and sunflower pack tremendous bang for your buck. And don't forget generous use of herbs and spices! These plant foods are positively vibrating with chi and loaded with antioxidants to combat fertility-blocking inflammation in both women and men.

Tune in to the vibrancy of fresh, energized vegetables and fruits, and it can even help you stay clear and open. Wise one Danica Thornberry says the clarity that comes from high-vibration food versus the dulling effect of overly refined or chemical-spiked foods is key to helping you hear the whisper of your spirit— and perhaps that of your child-to-be.

Fats and fertility go hand in hand. Hormones are made from cholesterol, which your liver does synthesize for you, yet most wise ones agreed that getting dietary cholesterol from healthy animal-food sources contributes to better hormone balance in their patients. Should you become pregnant, your baby's brain—among many other parts of her!—will flourish from the choline, omega-3 fatty acids, and fat-soluble vitamin A you provide from your real-food diet, so don't be shy about staying well fueled now with healthy saturated fats from clean sources—you'll see considerable use of grass-fed butter or ghee in my recipes—as well as cold-water fish, and whole-plant food fats—think coconut, avocado, nuts, seeds, and olives—as well as cold-pressed, unrefined oils made from those ingredients. Fats also support your immune system, combat inflammation, increase your warmth and circulation, and much, much more.

5. EXPERIENCE ALL FIVE FLAVORS

Traditional cooks from the East have always taken care to infuse the daily diet with the five flavors. In Ayurveda these are salt, sweet, sour, bitter, and astringent (astringent means drying, drawing fluids inward; think of the mouthfeel of a slightly unripe banana). Kerala's Dr. Venugopal says that all the tastes are necessary to bring the balance of the five elements—the fundamental forces of nature that combine into the doshas or bioenergetic influences determining your constitution and health. Each taste stimulates different activities in the body, and none is better or worse than the next; they are "equally good." TCM agrees, yet categorizes the tastes and their connection to the five main organ systems slightly differently: In addition to the Kidney-Salty and Spleen-Sweet connection, we have Liver-Sour, Heart-Bitter, and Lungs-Spicy/Pungent. Each flavor resonates with and supports each organ. The five flavors can also be used to address imbalances where they occur: salty can help dissolve stagnation;

PRECONCEPTION SUPPLEMENTS
AND HERBS

I believe that if you are committed to eating nutritious, fresh food every day—including the animal-sourced foods listed here—and your digestion is working well, you can get what you need from food. (Except for sufficient D_3—get it from sun exposure or be sure to supplement daily; see page 84.) If it proves challenging to hit the mark daily with your meals, consider using a high-quality multivitamin and a certified-pure omega-3 source (some like fermented cod liver oil, which contains vitamins A and D; others like krill oil) alongside. About three months before you hope to conceive, you could switch to a quality prenatal supplement, preferably food-based, or a brand recommended by a trusted practitioner, plus your omega-3s and additional vitamin D_3 as required. (Note: Seek out a prenatal that containes methylfolate, not folid acid.) Avoid the cheaper drugstore brands, which tend to be low-grade and contain fillers. If you feel called to use Chinese herbs, Women's Precious Pills and Free and Easy Wanderer are two formulas that can be safely used to repair, restore, and prepare in the three months prior to pregnancy.

sweet tonifies; sour calms; bitter clears heat; and spicy expels wind and cold. You don't have to be an Eastern-trained practitioner to use flavors to balance. Just listen. Dr. V says that your body will tell you which it needs if you pay attention to your palate and its desires for a burst of tart grapefruit or a few bites of salty manchego cheese. He says to add condiments to your meals, just like in his homeland of Southern India where sweet chutney and sour yogurt is heaped on a banana leaf to complement the spicy lentils and rice in the center. Think sauerkraut, salsa, or the yogurt and tartar sauces in the recipes that follow. I created the recipes in this book partly to expose your taste buds to new flavors, so please try the unusual ones—like sour dark vinegar, salty oysters, bitter dandelion, spicy pepper, or cilantro—even if you're not sure about them! It's also easy to find lists online of the foods that represent all five tastes. And as any chef will tell you, always remember that salt is your friend. A good Celtic sea salt, chock-full of oceanic minerals, helps to maintain your healthy balance of body fluids and keep your blood moving.

Last, remember to stay well hydrated. Water is essential for making healthy amounts of cervical mucus, as well as your mate's semen, his conduit for sperm. The old ways advise not going wild with water—guzzling too much can deplete your body of minerals. Consistent sipping, plus plenty of water-filled vegetables and fruits in moderation help you stay hydrated.

intuitive eating

Take inspiration from these five ideas and also listen in to what feels right to you. To my mind, the highest form of healthy eating is intuitive—knowing what you need, honoring the ebbs and flows. Sound easier said than done? You're probably already eating intuitively without realizing it. On a winter day, iceberg lettuce is not as appealing as roasted tomato soup; when spring's asparagus and artichokes appear, the craving hits for these clarifying foods drenched in olive oil and garlic. Over the months (or years!) of a preconception prelude, you'll naturally shift between a hunger for denser, building foods and lighter, clearing foods. Listen up and feed these body's urges! There's nothing to fear. When you arrive at a place where most of the ingredients in your kitchen are benevolent and when your digestion is working well, you can trust these bodily messages—they come from a good place. There's a saying: you crave what you eat. The more you eat simply prepared, whole foods, free of sugar and additives, the more you will crave that type of food. (One caveat: the midwife Davi Khalsa taught me that if you are craving sugars, your body almost always is asking for protein.)

Why does this relate to the woman's path, the mothering path in particular, you might ask? Because we are cyclical, not linear, as our wise ones have endlessly pointed out. Our energy, our outlook, our fortitude and our

FERMENTED FOODS

At MotherBees and in my home, small servings of fermented foods like sauerkraut and other cultured vegetables like kimchi, and miso and coconut kefir and yogurt, as well as drinks like kombucha, appear in many meals. We've all heard by now how probiotic-rich fermented foods contribute to healthier gut environments, helping our immune systems and letting us absorb more nutrition. From a traditional perspective, the sour tastes of many of these foods support the liver and because they use enzymatic activity to stimulate digestion, they move and direct the chi—which is vital to prevent stagnation and stay at your best.

sensitivity shift in different moments; we live in perpetual response to bigger cycles and rhythms. Yet the linear world we live in doesn't always honor that truth. Learning to listen in to what your organ systems are saying and then answering them with food is a gift you give yourself, especially when it comes to meeting the demands of becoming a mother. You might notice that you're feeling depleted, rundown, or out of gas and know that your Kidneys need some building foods. Or detect you're feeling weaker than normal, overwhelmed by too much to do, or even feeling as needy as a child, and you realize your Spleen needs softer, warmer, comforting fare—it's craving comfort and safety. And those moments when you're irritated beyond measure, quick to snap and react? You'll know what to do. Your Liver's asking for clearing foods, a break from anything clogging, a chance for release. This inner conversation doesn't have to be fluent, but when it's there, profound changes can occur. You can start to feel as if your body and you are in this together, no matter what—you're on the same team, through thick and thin. The bond gets stronger; you trust your body more. And you get a practice ground for mothering, through paying deep attention and responding to ever-changing needs. Intuitive eating teaches you to tend to yourself as kindly as you hope to one day tend to your child.

feeding your cycle

DANICA THORNBERRY shared her ideal foods for supporting yourself during your cycle, especially when you are actively seeking to conceive. Consider this a way in to a deeper listening to your body, and serving its subtle needs.

1 While you're bleeding, be sure to consume cleansing green plant foods, high in fiber and cellulose, to pull out unopposed toxic estrogens from the previous cycle, cooked lightly or in soups for warming effect. These iron-rich greens combine well with red meat to build the blood after your menstrual bleed.

2 In the second half of the follicular phase, support your recruiting and maturing follicles and the building up of estrogen levels with fat-rich foods like avocado, coconut, egg yolk, fatty fish like salmon and cod, and whole-fat dairy (preferably raw).

3 After ovulation and possible fertilization, enjoy foods that keep your body temperature warm and don't cause a lot of digestive distress. Butternut squash soup made with onions (not overly heating ginger), beef stew, chicken soup, bone broths, and curries, and sattvic Black Sesame Rice Porridge (page 201) will do the trick!

4 In the second half of your luteal phase, the week leading up to a pregnancy test or your period, help your blood sugar stay balanced with foods that have a low glycemic index value. Nix bread, refined carbs, and sugars and keep healthy trail mix on hand made of nuts and seeds, dried red fruits and berries (goji berries, cranberries, goldenberries aka "gooseberries," cherries) and sprinkle pomegranate seeds generously if in season. The nutrients in red berries help to nourish your blood, which is very important to keep the uterus lining thick during this time of possible implantation. Delight your senses with pops of color and flavor—you'll love feeling more balanced during this week of fluctuating hormones! ○

6

conceiving

The Ayurvedic doctor and botanical drug expert Dr. Jay Lokhande gives an unusual prescription to child-hopeful couples who come to him for guidance. Trained in Ayurveda's time-honored knowledge of the science of life, his advice starts with the pillars of a disciplined lifestyle, and ends somewhere higher: with intention and invocation. In Dr. Jay's tradition, having a child is a sacred act that transcends the simple mechanics of biology—it requires bringing your physical, mental, and spiritual selves to the process. To cultivate balance in body, mind, and spirit, he encourages couples to follow a holistically healthy lifestyle—much as we've outlined in the previous chapters—but as it gets closer to launch date, his instructions are a bit more specific, and a bit more spiritual.

He walks couples through a detailed conception ritual called *garb-hadhana* that springs from ancient teachings, but remains, he says, remarkably effective for couples today. The regimen begins seven days before any intimacy occurs and requires the daily ingestion of a "saatvic" or ojas-building rice porridge made from goat, almond, coconut, or camel's milk (good luck finding *that* in the fridge of your local grocer)—the woman's spiked with black sesame seeds to energetically resonate with, and stimulate, her eggs. (For a recipe, see page 201.) The couple will adhere to the avoidance of all meat products, and commit to a daily his-and-her practice of sitting back-to-back, invoking prana or spiritual life-force, and breathing together in harmony to subtly build the ojas (see the breathing practice in Chapter 4, Clearing, on page 119) in each and help them fall into gentle alignment. On the day of intercourse, an event that has been timed with the woman's ovulation schedule, the couple is to follow these steps to the letter: they should be ensconced at home by 5 P.M., stash away all their electronic devices, consume their porridge as soon as the sun goes down, and take a short rest from 9 P.M. to 11 P.M., all in preparation for the sacred act that will take place around midnight, the most fortuitous part of the evening. After that, they will breathe consciously together while praying to the spirit of their unborn child. It is at this point that they are finally ready to make love—in the missionary position only, as it represents mother as the earth and father as the sky. Then, as the man "releases his seed," he must exhale consciously—inhalation is life and exhalation is death and to birth something new, the old must first fade away. After, the mother lies on her back for at least forty-five minutes breathing consciously. The next morning the couple will cleanse their bodies from head to toe.

Not your average romp in the hay, is it?

Dr. Jay sees garbhadhana as the ideal combination of Ayurvedic science, romance, and spirituality. He knows that committing to becoming pregnant in this way is not as simple as getting tipsy on date night and jumping into bed, but the results make the effort worthwhile. When a couple follows a balanced, disciplined lifestyle and practices garbhadhana, he says, conception occurs 95 percent of the time within three to four cycles. That number can serve as an inspiring light as you tune in even deeper to the awakening mother stirring within you and move into the last chapter of this book—and possibly the final stage along the path to becoming pregnant. Whether you practice garbhadhana or not, tapping into the scientific-romantic-spiritual trifecta—within yourself and within your relationship with your partner—will hold you firmly at this stage of the journey. This means viewing conception first from a place of science. Once you've got the facts straight, you'll have a firm foundation from which to add the flourishing touches. Basically, having a clear understanding of the technicalities of baby making will help you make a baby. To make things easier, we've already explored the workings of your cycle in Chapter 3, Preparing, and here we take a closer look at the process of human fertilization, distilling it into a few (mind-blowing) points to give you some perspective as you dive into the actual act of creation.

what's really happening in there?

As you enter this concluding chapter of the book, we hope that you have a solid grasp of what's happening on your side of the reproductive street (if not, a quick review of Chapter 3, Preparing, can give you a necessary refresh) and are tracking your cycle—or are at least planning to start ASAP, to maximize the chances of "catching the egg." You are using one of the many apps available today, a highly accurate ovulation predictor device (we're excited about OvuSense), or even an old-school paper-and-pencil tracking system. You know when you're ovulating, with no delusions about how short a window you have each cycle.

STRESS: THE ENEMY OF OVULATION

When you feel the urge to become a mother, the call can be downright deafening. The only way to quiet the noise, it seems, is to become pregnant as quickly as possible. But contrary to the urgency you may feel, this is often not a switch that can simply be flipped. It's a process. To complicate matters further, the stress that's created from the desire to make it happen ASAP can interfere with the mechanics of every step, as you learned in Preparing, including the progesterone and immune-system balance required to support a viable pregnancy.

The solution? Commit to stress-free living—especially during the heightened days of ovulation. This may seem like an impossible ask given the finite nature of your fertile window and the high stakes that surround creating a human being, but your healthy pregnancy depends on it. Holding on to the sweetness, and the sacredness, that is at the heart of making a baby can help you avoid categorizing pregnancy as yet another anxiety-fueled deadline that you must not fail to meet.

Though you're an ever-evolving entity whose cycle can be influenced by illness, travel, and stress, generally you're working with about five fertile days a month. You have become increasingly adept at recognizing when those days are happening by following the information relayed by your cervical mucus. (In fact, you can finally say "mucus" without cringing because you get that it's the primary guide to understanding when you're fertile.) When your mucus is in peak form, with that tell-tale egg-white-y stretch, it's your sign that ovulation is imminent and it's time to get down to business. Experts agree that it's critical to have sex *before* ovulation occurs, in the lead-up days when mucus is abundant, and especially when it's at its peak, than when it dries up, because at that point it's too late.

Careful timing is doubly important if you're older, because cervical mucus tends to diminish as you age, making your fertile window smaller. The good news is that research shows that when a woman in her late thirties hones in on her window accurately, she has the same conception rate as a woman in her early twenties who is just slightly more relaxed about the timing of intercourse. Regardless of your age, when you're hoping to conceive, have sex at least every other day around ovulation, but not more than once in twenty-four hours, as too much sex can deplete jing/ojas and, according to Auntie Ou, make the "baby room" tired—you're looking for quality over quantity here. The herbalist Chad notes that the older men get, the less they should be releasing their seed—if they want potent seed. It's also important to avoid commercial lubricants as they are the wrong pH value and can make it hard for sperm to get where they're trying to go (if you really want some outside lubrication, use Pre-Seed, as it's designed to match fertile cervical mucus).

And what of the sperm who embark on the quest for the holiest of grails? About 200 million sperm cells are released when a man ejaculates, but the journey is arduous and only one fiercely strong and determined swimmer will make it to the promised land. Just 10 percent of the sperm that embark on this adventure will make it through the cervix, and fewer still make it up to the top of the uterus, an odyssey akin to a human being climbing Everest. Half the remaining sperm head to the empty fallopian tube. The others head in the right direction—toward the waiting egg—and they stop to enjoy a tiny rest and take in some fortification (i.e., nutrients found on the walls of the tube). Once recharged, they burst forward toward the newly released egg in a group that has been trimmed down to a few dozen. At this point, the remaining hearty sperm will gather around the egg, but only one will be granted entry into the egg's inner chambers, where fertilization will take place.

From here, if all goes well, the egg and sperm, now a one-celled entity called a zygote, will begin dividing into a cluster of cells and will travel back down the fallopian tube to the uterus, where it will implant in the uterine lining (at this stage it's a blastocyst) and get to its primary task: creating cells that will eventually become the embryo and the placenta. About twelve days after conception, placental blood circulation and hormone production kicks in, a marker that is usually detectable in a woman's urine by a home pregnancy test (cue excited shouts from the bathroom!). There are lots of ideas about the positions a woman can put herself in to increase the chances of conception and implantation—raising your legs after sex, standing on your head, and so on—but our wise ones keep their postcoital advice simple: After attempting to conceive it's best to stay put for ten to twenty minutes (postcoital tenderness, anyone?), and in the week after intercourse take a break from working out. That's it. Some gentle movement is good as it keeps blood and chi flowing, but higher-level exertion can interfere with implantation.

conception: the practical and poetic

Now, armed with the biological facts of conception, plus all the fertility apps, websites, and books a human could possibly ingest (it's okay, we're extreme researchers, too), you may be tempted to tackle the process of conceiving a baby with a scientist's precision. But just as the lead-up to conception has been about more than the workings of your body alone—your head and heart were a big part, too—so is conception itself. There is an invitation now to bring a level of sacredness, or at least some heart-fueled intention, to this concluding stage of the journey. Regardless of your belief system, it's pretty clear that making a baby is the greatest act of creation and therefore deserving of a certain level of reverence. Yet so many of us barrel into the experience forgetting that it is about so much more than biology. When you bring consciousness or awareness to the act, it can transform the experience from something that is merely physical to something that is downright mystical, as demonstrated by each thoughtful step of the garbhadhana ceremony. But in the vast conversation about fertility and conception we find that very little is said about the esoteric aspects of baby making. If the idea is expressed at all, it can seem woo-woo; after all, there is an undeniable physical equation that must be followed for conception to occur: egg plus sperm, etc. It's almost too easy to remain clinical about it all, neglecting to notice when desire tips into neurosis—when you're forcing instead of allowing: *My fertile window is here! Must have sex now!* The love, tenderness, and passion at the heart of conception can be quickly extinguished by temperature charts and fertility-app alerts. We forget what's really going on here.

If you're not a crystal-toting meditator who can say "conscious conception" without rolling your eyes, accessing this kind of sacredness may seem like a stretch. But it's really not. You can keep one foot comfortably planted in the realm of the physical, mastering the fluctuations of your own cycle and the mechanics of human reproduction, while simultaneously opening yourself up to the profound heart-expansion that is available every time you and your partner enter intimate space with the intention of conceiving a child. This is the middle path. To get there you simply need to be present to what's happening in the moment you're in rather than allowing yourself to be swept away into thoughts of what's going to happen in the future. To clarify, the future is any moment after the moment you're currently inhabiting—ten seconds from right now, ten months from now, and ten years from now are equally the future. If you're making love with your partner, do your best to stay there. Try not to think about how you'll feel when you take the pregnancy test in a few weeks or if your progeny will like ballet or baseball. We understand that the fierce longing for a baby can pose a very real challenge to remaining present, that it's way easier said than done. But there is an effective tool that is always available for you when it feels hard to be where you actually are.

When you find your mind spinning ahead of you, you can stop the cycle with your breath. Conscious breathing

How many people you know when "doing" conception can't conceive, and yet when they give up on conception, they conceive? There's a certain amount of open yin energy required to conceive. As much as we want our men to not be toxic masculine, we need them to be yang. As much as we want our women to be empowered, we need them to be yin and receptive—not too active and heady and doing. It comes together in what we call *wu wei* in TCM—a dance of effortless action.

—CHAD CORNELL

is like pushing the reset button. It calms the parasympathetic nervous system, changing your state of being from anxious and distracted to calm and receptive. Simply take three full breaths, in through the nose and out through the mouth, and bring your attention to your senses. Feel the heat of your partner's skin on yours, taste his lips, really look into his eyes. Pay radical attention to each other. This will shoot you back to the present moment and reconnect you both to what's driving you to come together in such open intimacy—the desire to create your child.

a grand purpose

Remaining present with your partner as you actively unite to create a child is another representation of the state of balance and harmony that is at the heart of awakening the fertility within you. When you shift the experience of conceiving a child from a rigid got-to-get-it-done accomplishment to an experience infused with levity and love, your heart will remain soft and open, leading to less stress and anxiety. Less stress supports every step of the conception process, before, during, and after. Plus, when you choose to come together with a shared intention of creating a baby, rather than a solo race against your ovulation clock, you fortify your relationship for whatever is to come. By consciously entering into the act of conception together, as two adults in harmony, you are signing an unwritten contract that says, "we both agree that we are ready to walk toward this next chapter." This requires belief in each other and faith that things will unfold as they are supposed to. It's as if you're holding hands and jumping off a cliff, not sure where exactly you'll land. By leaping into the unknown as a united front, you are establishing a foundation of trust that will carry you through any rocky waters that may be ahead—whether they are around conception, pregnancy, or parenting.

Like a hummingbird feeds off a flower, the man and woman savor the nectar of being in the presence of each other.

—CHAD CORNELL

Have you ever had a conversation with someone without actually talking? Maybe you're upset or excited and you're talking to that person in your head? Connecting with the spirit of your child is like that. You can simply sit quietly and open up to the spirit of the child you have not met yet. You can ask, simply, "Can I please hear the whispering of my baby's spirit, so I can understand how to serve him or her best?" —JAPA KHALSA

Our wise ones take it a step further. Many believe that sacredness is an unequivocal aspect of conception; that the man and woman who come together are serving a duty that surpasses the fulfilment of their own desire to have a child. By uniting with the hope to procreate, they are serving the soul of the being who wants to come into a physical body at this time. Japa Khalsa, our healer in New Mexico, sees the mother as a sacred vessel—by conceiving, carrying, and birthing a baby, she is transporting the heavens to the earth. The child's soul chooses the parents who will help it embody so it can live out its destiny. Making a baby takes on an entirely new dimension when viewed from this perspective! This is part of the reason Dr. Jay walks his clients through such an intentional conception ceremony. He aims to click them into the significance of what they're embarking upon from the outset—way before a baby is even in the picture. Parenthood is a life-altering, multilayered rite of passage that encompasses the entire range of human emotions, with currents of purpose and sacrifice running throughout. Entering into your role as parent with this awareness will help to give you the grace and resilience required for success.

Now, at the final phase, after months of pregnancy preparation, you are ready to step into a place of action and unite with your partner to create your child. As you enter that intimate space and breathe to remain grounded in the present moment, take note of your emotional state. Are you still coming from a goal-oriented place? If so, see if it's possible to shift your perspective a few degrees to touch into the sacredness of the agreement you are both making. Then go a bit deeper and clearly state that you are calling in the soul of your child. You can say it aloud to yourself or your partner, or silently to yourself. Either way, the intention will be there.

riding the waves

When hoping to become pregnant, there is a tendency to place a laserlike focus on your fertile days, completely forgetting that ovulation is one part of your cycle as a whole. During this time, your period can feel like a defeat. Menstruating was once a normal and expected part of your life, but now bleeding seems like a sign that you've failed in some way. These feelings are natural but not required. It is possible to loosen the grip on your ovulation calendar and lean into the wisdom of your cycle the way you did when you were busy preparing your body, mind, and spirit for conception. It is discouraging or disappointing (or just plain heartbreaking) to get your period after putting so much effort and intention to conceiving—a friend used to say that getting her period was like tears falling from the egg that didn't meet a sperm that cycle—but remember that your cycle is like the phases of the moon; it waxes and wanes. Your blood is a sign that it's time to regroup and rest. Holding the desire for a baby so deeply in your heart takes effort; regular, connected, conscious sex takes effort. Now is the time to pull back from all of that yang doing and sink into some yin being. There really isn't another option anyway. You've taken all the action that can be taken

Conceiving a child starts by asking, "What am I offering?" Consider how you will be giving back to the world by being a parent. Connect to the ways [in which] this act is your contribution to the greater good. When you cannot give anymore, your offspring will be able to.

—V.A. VENUGOPAL

The path you take to grow your family is uniquely yours. Some women may choose to pursue motherhood on their own; others may support the process with outside intervention like IVF or surrogacy; still others may pursue adoption or become a stepparent through marriage. Regardless of the path you take to get there, transitioning into this next chapter of your life from an awakened, aware state will nourish the sturdy ground that will hold you through the inevitable ups and downs that lie ahead. The heightened consciousness that a couple attains while coming together to make a baby can be applied to every iteration of becoming a mother. You do this by turning your attention, and intention, to the gateway you're about to walk through. If you're hoping to have a baby on your own, tap into the depth of what is happening—creating your child!—at every stage of the process; if you're adopting, feel the significance of bringing a new family member into your life; if you're using IVF, take time to connect to the soul of your child; and if you're becoming a stepmother, consider the significance of inheriting children to nurture and love.

for that particular cycle, and now it's time to pull your foot off the gas pedal and coast. Use this time to tend to those aspects of yourself that require attention— the parts of you that are *not* connected to baby making. Just because you are now actively intending to conceive, does not mean that you can stop nurturing your fertile life; it's actually more important than ever to be fulfilled and happy. Lacey Haynes, one of our wise ones in the United Kingdom, encourages you to ask a big question: Is your life something that a seed would want to be planted in? The latter half of your cycle, when your ovulation window has closed for the month, is the time to hone in on things that bring you joy and help you feel rested. Can you make time for yourself now?

sacred conception

AT WMN SPACE in Los Angeles, Paula Mallis supports women and their partners going through intense IVF procedures and surrogacy, as well as unmedicated conceptions. Though each story is different, there is a common current running through them all—a forgetting of the spiritual aspect of conception. Though a woman may be working with a trusted OB, as well as a fertility specialist and acupuncturist, and eating the right food, she can still feel lost, Mallis says. She attributes this empty feeling to the woman's need to form a relationship with the soul of her baby. Through gentle one-on-one guidance, and by holding a "loving, neutral place," Mallis helps them connect and dialogue with the soul of their baby. "Connecting with baby's spirit allows there to be a connection to more than what's happening on the physical level— it acknowledges the emotional and spiritual level, as well," she explains. This can be especially impactful for women who have been trying for years. There is a deep longing to connect with their baby and the process of communing with the baby's spirit can alleviate some of that longing.

In addition to the extra dimensions you now bring to lovemaking, consider adding another level of sacredness to the conception period. This can be with the intention to connect with your baby's spirit or to simply add an element of ritual to the experience. When you ritualize something, it helps you embark upon that thing with more presence. There is absolutely no wrong way to bring ritual into this time of conceiving. You and your partner can create your own version of the conception ceremony—sharing special words or phrases before getting intimate, breathing together while sitting facing each other, knee to knee, or bringing sacred objects into the room that represent your child or your growing family—natural elements like flowers or stones or perhaps a pair of baby booties (if they don't kill the mood). Or consider enhancing your boudoir with a statue of a pregnant woman or image of a mother holding a newborn (both said to enhance fertility). You can also create an altar with special items and sacred plants (sage, palo santo, sweet grass) that stands as an ongoing symbol of your desire to bring your child into the world. Even something as simple as lighting a special candle or reciting a short prayer before making love brings ritual, and sacredness, to the act. ⬡

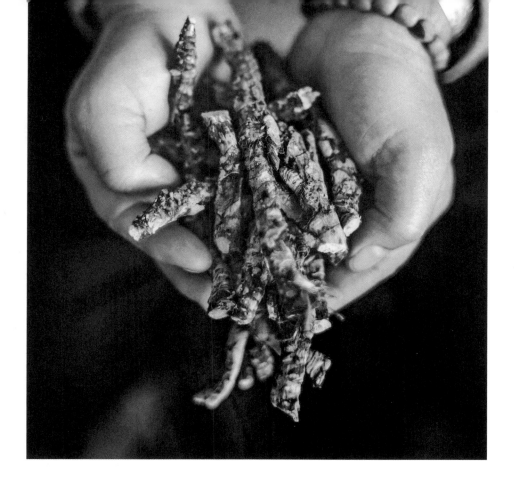

the surrender experiment

Throughout the pages of this book, we've asked you to turn your attention to preparing for pregnancy. We've shared practical information, and rejuvenating recipes, to fortify your body and a good amount of spiritual guidance to open your heart. At every stage of the process, the energy driving us to create this book has been strong—strong enough to pull us away from our kids and other breadwinning duties and attach us to our computers until we are delirious and bleary-eyed. As with *The First Forty Days*, we are driven to shine light on an essential stage of a woman's journey that has until now been relegated to the ranks of an afterthought—and to remind you that you are not alone. As you traverse the twists and turns along the road to pregnancy, some of them unexpected and some of them unwelcome, we hope that you will tap into the invisible but ever-present web of sisterhood that connects women everywhere. This connection is especially useful when things are hard. And they can get hard at some points. You may have checked all the boxes on your preparation checklist: eaten the right foods, tamed your stress, and taken inventory of your unprocessed hurts and fears, and yet conception still eludes you. You're not alone. Someone else is going through something similar right now—while others are going through a different set of challenges. We are all in our own chapter in our motherhood story, with our own histories and circumstances—some

A RED TENT DAY

Julia Barokov, coauthor Marisa's Buddhist-minded therapist, gives her female clients (some of whom are on the roller-coaster ride of getting pregnant, some of whom are managing PMS symptoms, others who are navigating the modern epidemic of overwhelm-induced anxiety) a clear assignment: take a red tent day. Inspired by Anita Diamant's iconic 1997 book, this is a full day of "you time," originally prescribed for the early phase of your cycle, during PMS and menstruation, but we encourage you also to consider giving yourself a red tent day in the second half of your cycle, when your ovulation window has closed and there's nothing to do but surrender to what will be. Truthfully, we wish you could take a red tent *month*—if you do, can we join?—but claiming one day a month just for yourself, to do nothing more than be gentle with yourself, is a strong start. Acceptable activities include getting a massage, reading a novel in a café, having lunch with a dear friend, or taking a walk in the woods. Unacceptable activities include running errands that can wait, doing chores you dislike, checking work emails, or reading anything connected to making a baby. You could spend your whole day napping, working on a creative project, or luxuriating at a spa. It's your day. Do what feels best—just be sure to put it on your calendar.

of us are older, some younger, some hoping to become mothers for the first time, others looking to expand their families—yet we are united by the great equalizer that is the mystery of creation. Try as we can to tame it or understand it, to apply science or spirit, the process is wild and miraculous and refuses to be confined by a set of rules or how-tos. There is no magic formula for getting pregnant—but the process is ultimately benevolent even if it doesn't feel like it right now. If you are faced with an unexpected outcome, perhaps an inability to get pregnant or one or more miscarriages, there may be a massive gift tucked inside all that hurt. This is not some hokey silver-lining talk. This is real life. When you muster the courage to truly surrender to what is happening, to let go and accept what actually *is* (not what it should be, what you want it to be, or what it once was) with all of its searing pain and discomfort, you open yourself up to great beauty and wisdom, ultimately awakening to who you really are. This is some of the deepest emotional work you'll do in a lifetime.

Awakening your fertility is a journey. For some it's an uncharted expedition with unexpected twists and turns, dark tunnels, and shaky bridges. Though your heart may hold a clear desire to mother a child, the process that leads you there may end up illuminating parts of yourself that are crying out for their own version of mothering. This is a good thing. We wrote this book so that every new recipe you make, every hard conversation you have, and every healthy habit you establish, will fortify your body, strengthen your resolve, soften your heart, and calm your mind—this is a deep tending to yourself. The path to becoming a mother is a mystery. It is impossible to predict when you'll get pregnant or how. You can't know what your child will look like or be like or how parenthood will influence your relationship with your partner. But you can be ready for anything that lies ahead by becoming the most whole version of yourself that you can be.

Wherever you are on your road to motherhood, whether it's a far-off dream or a reality you wish to manifest right now, use the three universal insights as your guideposts along the way.

CONSERVE YOUR FERTILITY POTENTIAL by tending to the three organ systems (Kidney, Liver, Spleen) through harmonious lifestyle choices, stress release, and deeper listening to the subtle, and not-so-subtle, messages of your body. Your fertility potential is an expression of your state of jing or ojas and noticing how you feel in any given moment can relay key information about how much of the precious essence you are expending. Are you depleted, irritated, or overwhelmed? Commit to following the bread-crumb clues provided by your state of being. The more fluent you get in the language of your body, the easier it will be to meet its ever-changing requirements.

FILL YOUR RESERVES before actively attempting to become pregnant. Start by removing the bad stuff, the processed, packaged, and manufactured foods (junk foods, party foods, overindulgent foods, and alcohol, of course) and move toward wholesome, colorful, unprocessed foods, free from chemicals and preservatives. The goal is to become deeply nourished, but to pursue it with a light touch, as your digestive system functions optimally when you are relaxed and happy, allowing you to get the most out of the good food you're consuming.

LET YOURSELF BLOOM! As you travel toward the dream of motherhood, be sure to hold on to the moment-to-moment treasures that you encounter along the way. Each time you laugh with a friend, stop to smell a flower, or gaze into a pair of eyes you love, you are making a deposit in your spiritual bank account and fortifying the soil of your fertile life. The

> If raising children is a woman's life purpose, then nothing is going to stand in the way of her getting there. I help her fall into faith and trust that there is something way bigger than her. If she comes in catastrophizing, I help her gain perspective and reframe. I help her to know that her path is unfolding, that she is on a path that is leading her somewhere.
>
> —DANICA THORNBERRY

rewards are twofold: you remain present in the life you are living right now, rather than giving it away to the longing for something that's not here yet, and you pave the way for an easeful conception and a healthy pregnancy by remaining open and receptive—positively yin-ified, if you will. So, take walks in nature, make lots of love (as much as you can, make love to make love, not to make a baby), and connect with others. If partnered, stay close to each other emotionally. Practice vulnerability by having the real—often hard—conversations. We are wired to crave genuine belonging and understanding and can only receive it if we are honest about who we are and what we are feeling. Take a risk and be real. Then zip it and listen.

Connect with women. Keep the current that unites us active and alive. Talk to your mother about her experiences surrounding conception, pregnancy, and birth. Ask about your grandmother's. Share your most tender thoughts with your girlfriends—are you afraid, angry, uncertain, or hopeful? Then make room for them to share theirs. Awakening your fertility is your unique journey, but you don't have to do it alone. We need each other. And just as our wise ones generously passed their teachings on to us so we could pass them on to you, please pass this book to the women in your life.

RELAX INTO YOUR ESSENCE

Ulrike Remlein, our healer in Germany, shares a sentiment with every woman who is actively inviting in conception. She asks you to trust that you are love. Whether you conceive in that cycle, she reminds you to trust there is a reason, and that what's most important is to practice relaxing back into your being, your very essence, and to know that all is well. "The best place to be," counsels Ulrike, "is in deep acceptance of what is."

7

recipes

PROTEINS

The prelude to pregnancy is a season of fortifying your body. Add slow-cooked stews, simply prepared fish, warming beans, and quick-hit one-bowl dishes to your repertoire, and you'll find that feeding yourself and your beloved—and any children already in your life—doesn't have to take excess effort or thought. Keep an eye out for the jing-supporting foods scattered throughout—seaweed, nuts and seeds, healthy fats, and a touch of organ meat.

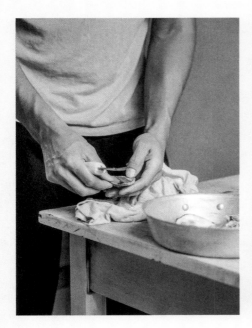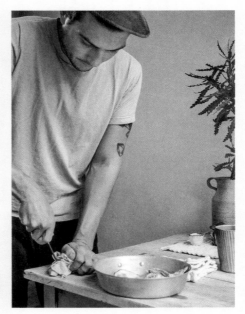

Oyster Fritters, page 174

hearty bean stew with kombu and walnuts

SERVES 4

This filling stew is a Kidney-building power-house. Deep-hued kidney beans are the star; jing-preserving and thyroid-supporting kombu seaweed is the support player (it also reduces gas from the beans); and then there's a secret ingredient: walnuts, pureed so finely that they lend a depth of flavor and a creamy texture that will get people wondering what kitchen tricks you have up your sleeve. Use your choice of broth, vegetable or bone, and give yourself a pat on the back. You've created a super-nourishing bowl.

2 cups (370 g) dry red kidney beans

1 dry kombu strip

4 cups (960 ml) cold filtered water

½ (65 g) cup roughly chopped walnuts

2 tablespoons ghee

½ cup (25 g) peeled and diced carrots

1 cup (150 g) diced yellow onion

½ cup (90 g) diced red bell pepper

2 cloves garlic, coarsely chopped

1 teaspoon sweet paprika

2 teaspoons coriander seeds

6 cups (1.4 L) low-sodium vegetable or bone broth

¼ cup (60 ml) extra-virgin olive oil

Sea salt and black pepper

½ cup (15 g) roughly chopped parsley, for garnish

In a medium pot, soak the dry red kidney beans and dried kombu in 3 cups (720 ml) cold filtered water. In a small bowl, soak the chopped walnuts with 1 cup (240 ml) cold filtered water. Leave both covered loosely with plastic wrap in the fridge overnight, for at least 8 hours.

The next day, warm the ghee in another medium pot over medium heat. Add the carrots, onion, red bell pepper, and garlic. Cook, stirring periodically, until the vegetables begin to caramelize, about 10 minutes. Add the paprika and coriander seeds and cook for an additional 2 minutes, or until they become aromatic.

Add the strained red kidney beans, wet kombu strip, and broth, bringing the liquid to a boil over medium-high heat. Once the liquid starts to boil, bring the heat down to medium-low and simmer, covered, for 45 minutes to 1 hour, until the liquid is reduced by about 20 percent, then leave uncovered. Check the beans periodically for tenderness. You can add more broth or water if the liquid cooks down quicker than anticipated or the kidney beans need more cooking time.

While the beans are cooking, strain the walnuts. Combine the walnuts and olive oil in a blender and puree until very smooth. Once the kidney beans are soft, stir in the walnut puree. Season with sea salt and black pepper. Serve warm, garnished with the parsley.

TIP You may substitute coconut oil for the ghee if you like, though do give ghee a try. Grass-fed ghee, made by cooking off the milk proteins in butter until only the fat remains, is full of fat-soluble vitamins and a unique blend of short-, medium-, and long-chain fatty acids with healing and rejuvenating qualities. A sattvic food that helps build ojas, golden ghee is a gem of Ayurvedic cooking.

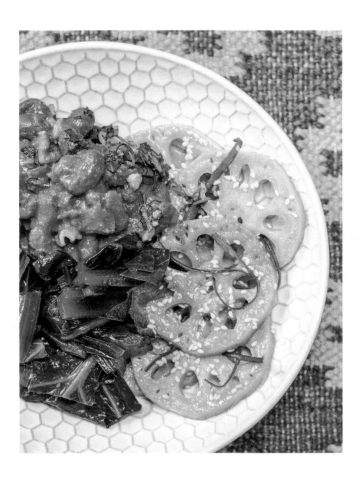

Prep time: 15 minutes, plus 8 hours soaking   Cook time: 1 hour

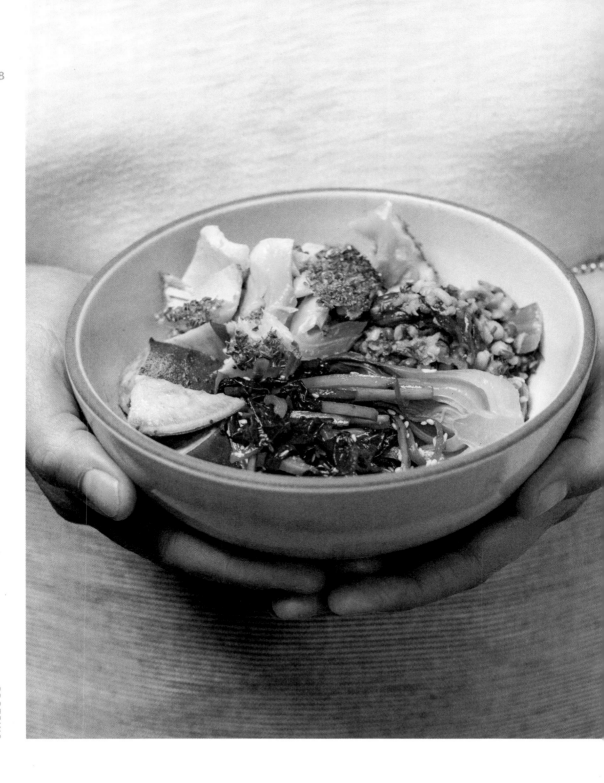

fennel-and-coriander-crusted wild salmon

SERVES 4

Wild salmon gets a permanent place at the preconception table thanks to its superb nutritional value. With its vibrant orange-pink color, it's also a delight to the senses. This preparation has you toast and grind spices—a traditional technique that releases the aromas like nothing you've experienced before!—to make a wonderfully flavored, crunchy crust that balances the salmon's creamy texture. The spices serve an extra purpose: coriander is warming and fennel supports the digestive fire.

¼ cup (20 g) whole coriander seeds

2 tablespoons whole fennel seeds

4 (2- to 3-ounce per serving) wild salmon fillets

Sea salt and black pepper

3 tablespoons grass-fed butter

1 teaspoon maple syrup (optional)

½ lemon

Heat a medium pan over medium-high heat and toast the coriander and fennel seeds for 2 minutes, or until they get very aromatic. When they are toasted, pour the seeds into a mortar and grind them with a pestle until they break, leaving them chunky rather than finely ground—you are not looking for a powder.

TIP If you don't have a mortar and pestle, place the spices on a cutting board and press the bottom of a pan on the seeds until they break.

Next, wash the salmon fillets and pat dry with a paper towel. Season each fillet with salt and pepper on both sides, and then coat the flesh side with the crushed-spice mixture by placing the spices on a plate and lightly pressing the fillets down into the mixture.

Melt the butter in a large stainless-steel pan over medium heat. When the butter starts to smoke slightly, place the salmon fillets in the pan spice side down. Lower the heat to medium-low and cook the fillets for 7 to 9 minutes, depending on how done you like your salmon.

Once there is a light-brown layer and three-quarters of the salmon is light pink, flip the salmon and lower the heat. Pour the maple syrup, if using, over the salmon (it will run down and caramelize the bottom) and cook for another 2 to 3 minutes, using a spoon to baste the spice side of the salmon with warm butter. When you press down on the salmon with your fingers, the flesh should bounce back immediately.

Finish with a squeeze of lemon juice.

Prep time: 15 minutes   Cook time: 15 minutes

PROTEINS

pork and kabocha squash stew

SERVES 6

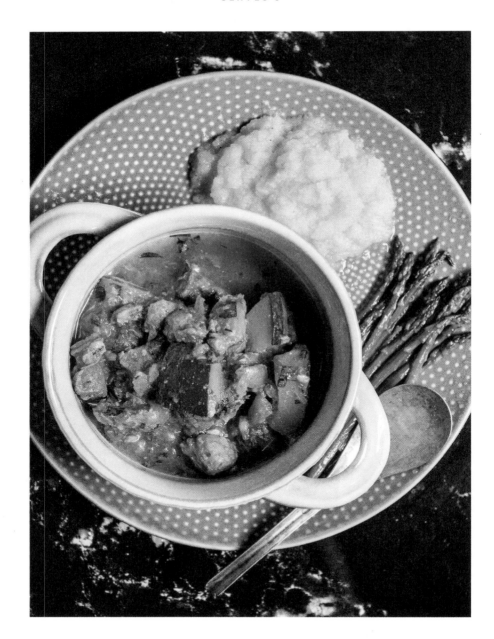

I've made this super-satisfying stew countless times, and scraped-clean bowls always get presented for seconds. The secret is in the harmony of flavors and textures: rich pork, meaty kabocha squash, and a gentle hit of circulation-enhancing chili merge as the stew slow cooks and fills the kitchen with mouthwatering whispers of what's to come. Serve with a heaping side of cooked greens and be generous with the nutrient-filled toppings—it can all fit in one bowl if you choose!

In a mixing bowl, combine the pork, coriander powder, garlic, and pinch of sea salt. Fold the ingredients together with your hands or a spoon. Cover the bowl with plastic wrap and refrigerate for 1 hour.

Heat the avocado oil in a large pot over medium-high heat. Take the pork out of the fridge and brown all sides of the cubes in small batches. (If you stack the pork, the sides will not brown.) Set aside the browned pork in a dish.

In the same pot, add the red chili flakes, onions, oregano, pork, and cold filtered water. Bring the liquid to a boil, then reduce to a simmer over medium-low heat, cover, and cook for roughly 1 to 1½ hours, until the pork is tender. Periodically skim the top layer of fat and discard with a ladle or a spoon and stir.

About 30 minutes before the pork is tender, add the kabocha squash to the pot and simmer until the squash is fork-tender and the liquid is a thick stew.

Add the chopped cilantro and pumpkin seeds when serving.

3 pounds (1.4 kg) pork shoulder, cut into 1-inch (2.5 cm) cubes

½ teaspoon coriander powder

2 cloves garlic, coarsely chopped

Sea salt

2 tablespoons avocado oil

Pinch red chili flakes

2 yellow onions, peeled and roughly chopped

1 tablespoon dried oregano

10 cups (2.4 L) cold filtered water

1 medium kabocha squash, halved, seeds removed, and cut into 1-inch (2.5 cm) cubes (skin on)

1 cup (50 g) finely chopped cilantro

¼ cup (30 g) pumpkin seeds

Prep time: 1 hour   Cook time: 2 hours

motherbees beef bolognese

SERVES 6

Some days call for a grounding, nourishing bowl of steaming Bolognese. This quick version comes with a twist: chicken liver sneaking in, barely noticeable, to powerfully fill your reserves, and shiitake mushrooms adding extra layers of flavor and umami taste, making it seem as if the Bolognese has simmered for hours. Serve over Roasted Spaghetti Squash (page 186) or your favorite kind of pasta.

2 tablespoons extra-virgin olive oil or avocado oil

1 yellow onion, diced

Sea salt and black pepper

1½ pounds (680 g) organic ground beef, 90% lean/10% fat

½ stalk celery, diced

1 carrot, diced

2 brown shiitake mushrooms, destemmed, diced

2 cloves garlic, thinly sliced

1 (32-ounce) jar tomato sauce

2 pieces (40 g total) organic chicken liver, cleaned, finely chopped

1 teaspoon maple syrup (optional)

Heat the oil in a large pan over medium-high heat. Cook the onion with a pinch of sea salt; stir, turning down the heat to medium-low after the first 10 minutes. Cook for another 20 minutes—you will notice a light brown stickiness on the onion and pan. The natural sugars from the onion will eventually create a golden-brown color with additional rich flavors. Add the ground beef and stir once the meat begins to brown on one side, 5 to 10 minutes.

Add the celery, carrot, shiitakes, and garlic and sauté for 5 minutes. Add the tomato sauce and bring the mixture to a light simmer. Reduce the heat to medium and simmer for another 30 minutes, or until the sauce reaches a desired thickness, the vegetables are tender, and the flavors meld together.

In the last 10 minutes, stir in the chopped chicken liver. If you desire a slightly sweeter sauce, add the maple syrup and stir.

Season with sea salt and black pepper to taste.

TIP Dishes with liver can feel especially replenishing on the heavier days of your menstrual cycle. They're also incredibly fortifying for your partner. Reproductive potential gets a powerful boost from the weekly consumption of grass-fed or pasture-raised liver.

PROTEINS

Prep time: 15 minutes   Cook time: 90 minutes

trout with broccoli rabe

SERVES 4

Cooking a light white fish can feel intimidating, as if only a skilled chef can get it just right. Not so! This preparation pairs delicate white-fish flavor with the slightly bitter taste of broccoli rabe, and quickly delivers a full complement of nutrition on one plate—protein, omega-3 fats, multivitamins, minerals, and more. If you can't find trout, substitute branzino or any other light white fish. If broccoli rabe isn't available, baby broccoli (broccolini) or broccoli works well, too. Try serving it with Seasonal Veggie Succotash (page 188) and Nutty Green Yogurt Sauce (page 190).

2 whole rainbow trout, gutted, skin on

Extra-virgin olive oil

Sea salt and black pepper

1 clove garlic, thinly sliced

1 bunch broccoli rabe, ends cut off

Chili flakes

½ cup (120 ml) cold filtered water or broth of choice

Juice of ½ lemon

3 whole Brazil nuts, roughly chopped

Under cold running water, rinse the trout inside and out, then pat dry the insides and outsides with paper towels. Rub olive oil on the skin evenly and finish with a pinch of sea salt, skin and flesh side. Heat 3 tablespoons oil in a large nonstick pan over medium-high heat. Once the oil begins to smoke, slowly lower the trout into the oil, being careful not to splash it. Reduce the heat to medium and cook the trout for 7 to 10 minutes without moving it. When you notice a crispy skin and golden-brown color, gently flip the trout. Allow the trout to cook on the second side for another 7 to 10 minutes, until the same golden-brown color is achieved. Transfer the trout to a plate covered with a paper towel.

In a medium nonstick pan, heat 1 tablespoon oil over medium-high heat. Toast the garlic until it begins to brown. Add the broccoli rabe, pinch of chili flakes, and water or broth, then cover immediately. Once the liquid is evaporated and the broccoli rabe is tender, finish it with the lemon juice and chopped Brazil nuts and season with sea salt and black pepper to taste.

TIP When shopping for broccoli rabe, look for vibrant green stalks and ends that are freshly cut.

PROTEINS

Prep time: 10 minutes   Cook time: 15 minutes

oyster fritters

SERVES 4

Oysters are a renowned fertility food—
they fortify the Kidneys and their high
levels of zinc support healthy sperm and
eggs. My aunties say they help produce a Y
chromosome; myth or reality, the three dozen
oysters consumed before my son's conception
may have had an effect! Fritters are a fast
way to prepare them and give an extra
preconception boost with the fats in the eggs
and lard (a nutrient-rich fat that tolerates
high-heat cooking). Serve with Tartar Sauce
(page 191) and a salad.

16 medium fresh raw
   oysters

Cold filtered water

Juice of 1 lemon

½ cup (60 g)
   cornstarch

3 whole eggs, beaten

2 cups (175 g) panko
   bread crumbs,
   regular or gluten-
   free

2 tablespoons lard or
   butter

Sea salt and black
   pepper to taste

Shuck the oysters. Place the oysters in a bowl
of cold filtered water to rinse off grit or shell
shards, and set them aside on a large plate.

Pour the lemon juice over the oysters and
marinate for 10 minutes, then pat dry the
oysters on a plate with paper towels.

While the oysters are marinating, set up your
breading station: one bowl with the cornstarch,
a second bowl with the eggs and 1 tablespoon
water whisked together, and a third bowl with
the panko bread crumbs.

Dunk each oyster first into the cornstarch,
then into the egg mix, and finally into the
panko, coating evenly on both sides in
each step.

Melt the lard or butter in a nonstick pan
over high heat and fry each oyster for 3 to
5 minutes on each side. Place the fritters on a
plate covered with a paper towel, season with
sea salt and black pepper, and eat them hot.

TIP If you choose to consume raw oysters, take
some time to find the best source, keeping in mind
that oysters are freshest in the cooler months, from
September to April. You can easily make your own
mignonette sauce by combining red wine vinegar
or sherry vinegar, minced shallots, and salt to
taste. Or go the classic route by adding a squeeze
of fresh lemon or a dollop of cocktail sauce to
each raw oyster.

PROTEINS

Prep time: 20 minutes   Cook time: 15 minutes

lamb and lentil stew with chinese cabbage

SERVES 4

Chinese cabbage, also called napa cabbage, was a constant in my grandmother's kitchen—she would drop handfuls of the leafy yellow-green veggie into her soups and stews to ensure we consumed plenty of the cruciferous vegetable. In this warming, fortifying stew, cinnamon and raisins balance the occasionally gamey flavor of lamb or, if you'd rather, grass-fed beef. Enjoy it on its own or spooned over rice.

1 teaspoon cinnamon powder

Sea salt and black pepper to taste

1 pound (455 g) boneless leg of lamb or grass-fed beef or chuck roast, cut into 2-inch (5 cm) chunks

3 tablespoons avocado oil

2 carrots, peeled, cut into 1-inch (2.5 cm) pieces

1 celery stalk, cut into 1-inch (2.5 cm) pieces

1 clove garlic, roughly chopped

3 tablespoons tomato paste

8 cups (2 L) low-sodium beef or veggie broth

½ cup (100 g) green lentils

2 tablespoons golden raisins

2 cups (250 g) Chinese cabbage (cut into 2-inch/ 5 cm pieces)

¼ cup (15 g) chopped cilantro

Using your hands, massage the cinnamon powder and 1 teaspoon sea salt into the meat chunks in a medium mixing bowl. Cover with plastic wrap and place the bowl in the fridge for 1 hour. While the meat is marinating, prepare the rest of the ingredients.

After the meat is marinated, heat a large pot over medium-high heat, then add the avocado oil. When the oil begins to smoke slightly, add the meat, spreading it evenly on the bottom of the pot to brown. We are looking for the meat to brown evenly, so limit the stirring, especially in the first 5 minutes.

Add the carrots and celery and cook for 10 minutes, or until they become translucent. Add the garlic and stir everything together for 2 minutes. Stir in the tomato paste and broth and simmer over medium-low heat for 45 minutes.

Add the green lentils and golden raisins, then continue cooking for an additional 30 minutes.

During the last 10 minutes, add the Chinese cabbage, then add the cilantro and season to taste with sea salt and black pepper.

PROTEINS

Prep time: 1 hour   Cook time: 2 hours

shiitake mushroom and turkey stir-fry

SERVES 4

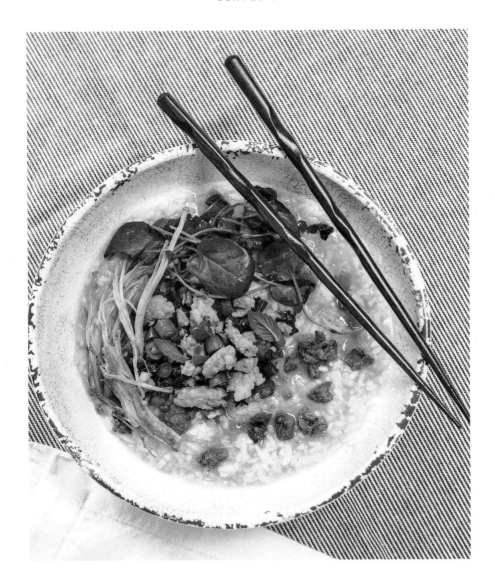

Prep time: 15 minutes   Cook time: 20 minutes

Few things bring me more pleasure in the kitchen than landing on the perfect bowl that combines a clutch of great ingredients into one simple serving. This vegetable-rich, high-protein, and umami-flavored concoction has become a MotherBees classic. Cruciferous cabbage, vitality-filled sprouts, immunity-building shiitake, and nourishing turkey are tossed in an addictive sauce that you'll be able to use on all kinds of improvised stir-frys once you've got it down.

In a small bowl, mix all the sauce ingredients. Set aside.

In a large nonstick pan over medium-high heat, add 1 tablespoon of the avocado oil. When it begins to smoke slightly, add the remaining 1 tablespoon avocado oil, the shiitake mushrooms, onion, ground turkey, garlic, carrot, and celery, being careful not to stack them too much. Sauté for 8 to 10 minutes, until the ingredients begin to brown, then add the sauce. Cook with the sauce for another 5 minutes, or until the sauce is reduced by half.

Remove the pan from the heat, add the green cabbage and bean sprouts, and mix together using tongs.

Top with the pumpkin seeds and green onion to serve. Season to taste with sea salt and black pepper.

TIP Substitute spinach or chard on days you don't feel like eating sprouts and green cabbage.

Sauce
¼ cup (60 ml) cold filtered water

¼ cup (60 ml) low-sodium tamari

⅛ teaspoon cane sugar (optional)

2 tablespoons sesame seeds

2 tablespoons rice vinegar

1 tablespoon mirin rice wine

2 teaspoons pure sesame oil

Stir-fry
2 tablespoons avocado oil

4 shiitake mushrooms, destemmed, sliced

¼ yellow onion, thinly sliced

1 pound (455 g) ground turkey

2 cloves garlic, roughly chopped

1 carrot, julienned

1 celery stalk, julienned

1 cup (100 g) shredded green cabbage

½ cup (50 g) bean sprouts

2 tablespoons pumpkin seeds

1 green onion, thinly sliced

Sea salt and black pepper to taste

six-flavor chicken

SERVES 4

Inspired by Southeast Asian street food, this super-flavorful ground chicken "crumble" has a hundred and one uses! It delivers a quick hit of protein and can be served so many ways—on a bowl of congee or well-cooked grains, on a salad, or even in tacos or lettuce wraps with added vegetables and pickles. I make a big batch and store it in an airtight container in the fridge. Dial the chili level up or down if you like—the touch of sugar helps to soften the heat.

2 tablespoons sesame oil

1 pound (455 g) ground chicken

1 cup (150 g) halved green beans

¼ teaspoon cane sugar

Pinch chili flakes

Pinch dried oregano

2 teaspoons oyster sauce

1 clove garlic, coarsely chopped

2 fresh basil leaves, thinly sliced

1 teaspoon freshly ground white or black pepper

Heat the sesame oil in a large sauté pan over medium heat and add the ground chicken. Sauté until cooked with a light brown color, roughly 10 minutes.

Add the green beans, cane sugar, chili flakes, and oregano and cook for an additional 5 minutes.

Add the oyster sauce and chopped garlic and cook for another 5 minutes. Top the dish with the basil and pepper of choice.

Prep time: 15 minutes   Cook time: 20 minutes

VEGETABLES

Fertility and whole-body vitality flourish when your diet is filled with fresh, energy-filled vegetables. Establish a die-hard habit of including them with every single meal, and snack on them, too. Pre-pregnancy is a time to discover just how many ways there are to cook vegetables, so you don't just default to noshing on chilly lettuce or tomatoes right out of the fridge. At MotherBees, we've landed on some classics for overall hormonal health. I've included a few wild cards here to make the exploration more exciting—have fun discovering some new ingredients and techniques.

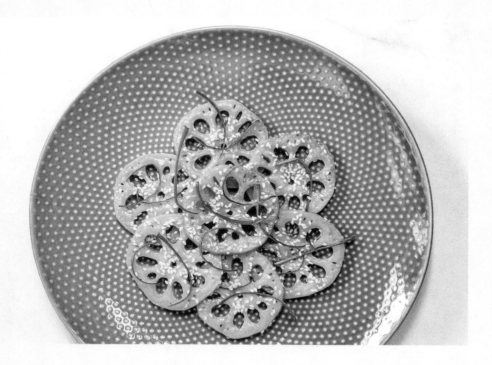

maple lotus root with pork

SERVES 4

At first glance, this dish may seem exotic, and yes, lotus root, longan fruit, and black vinegar might take a little sourcing. The results are worth it! Cooked lotus root has a sweet, crunchy, warm quality, and strengthens digestion, nourishes the blood, and tonifies chi. It's also so pretty and delicate-looking—it's seen as a symbol of purity and divine beauty! Slow-cooking pork bones creates a delicious broth that infuses the root with fortifying saturated fats and collagen, nourishing the Kidneys, supporting the adrenals, and soothing and repairing the intestinal wall so you can absorb the maximum nutrition from your food.

In a large pot over high heat, bring the cold filtered water, pork feet bones, and star anise to a quick boil. Skim any foam off the top and discard. Once the water comes to a boil, add the dried longan fruit, red dates, black vinegar, and lotus root and cook uncovered for 1 hour over medium-low heat.

Once the liquid is 75 percent reduced, stir in the maple syrup and taste the liquid. The liquid should leave your lips sticky and taste of caramelized maple.

Season with sea salt.

TIP Fresh lotus root can be found in most Chinese grocery stores. As an alternative, you can use water chestnuts. These can be found either fresh or sometimes packed raw in water in the ethnic or specialty aisles of grocery stores.

8 cups (2 L) cold filtered water

1 pound (455 g) pork feet bones, cut into 2-inch (5 cm) pieces

2 star anise pods

¼ cup (30 g) dried longan fruit (long yan rou)

¼ cup (45 g) whole red dates (dried jujube)

¼ cup (60 ml) black vinegar

2 fresh medium bulbs lotus root, peeled, sliced into ¼-inch (6 mm) rounds

1 tablespoon maple syrup

Sea salt

Prep time: 15 minutes   Cook time: 2 hours

trio of braised greens

SERVES 4

If there's one color you want to get really familiar with in the prelude to pregnancy, it's dark green. Dark leafy green vegetables are your absolute ally, helping build your reserves of folate and calcium, and moreover, they deliver essential nutrients to the liver so it can detoxify and balance hormones. They fortify the blood with iron and get your chi, your vital energy, absolutely dancing. At MotherBees, we collect armfuls of whatever dark greens are overflowing at the farmers' market, then cook them as follows. I hope you will enjoy these as often as we do!

1 tablespoon grass-fed butter or ghee

1 clove garlic, thinly sliced

½ bunch collard greens, deveined, cut into 2-inch (5 cm) pieces

½ bunch red chard, deveined, cut into 2-inch (5 cm) pieces

½ bunch spinach, cut into 2-inch (5 cm) pieces

2 cups (480 ml) low-sodium stock of choice

Sea salt, sesame seeds, and black pepper to taste

Warm the butter in a large pot over medium heat. Add the sliced garlic and stir frequently with tongs until the edges become light brown, about 3 minutes.

Add the collard greens and red chard and cook for another 5 minutes. Add the stock and reduce the heat to medium-low. Cover and let it all cook for 20 minutes, stirring periodically.

Add the spinach and cook covered for another 5 to 7 minutes. Add more liquid if the greens are not tender to your liking.

Season with sea salt, sesame seeds, and black pepper.

TIP   Definitely stir in heaps of dandelion greens if they're in season. This bitter green supports bile production, helping to move toxins and used-up hormones out of your intestines and begin to restore balance to menstrual cycles and relieve cramping that may be caused by a sluggish, overworked Liver.

VEGETABLES

coconut mashed sweet potato

SERVES 4

Creamy, dense, and satisfying, this earthy dish is the ultimate comfort food. Laced with dreamy fats, it's one of the easiest ways to show your Spleen some love (the fats also ensure you absorb beta-carotene and other micronutrients from this brightly colored food). Served with Trio of Braised Greens (page 181), it can fulfill a yearning for a lower protein, plant-based meal. Do try to find ume plum vinegar—made from Japanese umeboshi plums, this vinegar adds a surprisingly refreshing tart and salty-sweet flavor. It's a digestive tonic known to soothe the belly, clear toxins, and increase energy. Start with just a couple of dashes and discover its taste.

Cover the sweet potatoes with cold filtered water in a medium pot and place over medium-high heat. Bring the water to a boil, then lower the heat to medium. Let the sweet potatoes simmer until they are tender, about 20 minutes. Turn off the heat, drain the sweet potatoes, then place them back into the pot.

Add the coconut oil, butter or ghee, and ume plum vinegar, if using, then mash with a potato masher or a fork.

Season to taste with sea salt if not using ume plum vinegar.

3 cups (750 g) sweet potatoes (peeled, cut into 2-inch/ 5 cm cubes)

6 cups (1.4 L) cold filtered water

2 tablespoons coconut oil

2 tablespoons grass-fed butter or ghee

2 to 3 dashes ume plum vinegar (optional)

Sea salt, if not using ume plum vinegar

Prep time: 10 minutes   Cook time: 20 minutes

mung bean stew with bacon and bok choy

SERVES 4

You've had a long day. You know you should eat healthfully, but the takeout menu is calling. Turn to this recipe, which delivers maximum nutrition for minimal prep time (if you've established the habit of soaking your mung beans in advance, that is!). I adore mung beans—these tiny, gas-free beans are easy to digest, packed with folate, B_6, calming magnesium, and some protein. The bacon or pancetta adds some extra pre-pregnancy nutritional heft, and generous portions of bok choy ensure your plate brims with cleansing vegetables. Serve with well-cooked grains or even just mashed avocado.

2 tablespoons avocado oil

1 cup (250 g) smoked bacon (cut into small strips), or pancetta cubes (optional)

½ cup (75 g) diced yellow onion

2 cloves garlic, finely chopped

1 cup (200 g) mung beans, soaked overnight in cold filtered water, then drained

3 cups (720 ml) cold filtered water, or broth of choice

8 baby bok choy, quartered lengthwise

Sea salt and black pepper

Heat the avocado oil in a small pot over medium heat. Add the bacon strips and brown them, about 5 minutes.

Next, add the onion and cook until it becomes translucent and slightly caramelized.

Add the garlic, mung beans, and cold filtered water or broth and bring to a simmer. Cook for 30 minutes, or until the skin of the beans begins to split and become tender.

Last, add the bok choy, cover the pot, and cook for an additional 7 to 10 minutes, stirring periodically with a large spoon, until the bok choy becomes tender.

Season to taste with sea salt and black pepper.

VEGETABLES

Prep time: 15 minutes   Cook time: 45 minutes

sesame garlic asparagus

SERVES 4

Spears of asparagus shoot up through the earth announcing spring is here—a season of renewal and reinvigoration after the slower, heavier season of winter. No wonder its astringent qualities help clear the body of toxins and ama, cutting through any gunk. It's also a sperm-enhancing superstar, packed with nutrients that boost sperm quality. This is my favorite way to prepare it—garlic, broth, and sprinkles of yin-nourishing white sesame seeds decorating it like early spring flowers.

1 tablespoon extra-virgin olive oil or avocado oil

1 clove garlic, thinly sliced

1 bunch asparagus, ends cut off, halved

½ cup (120 ml) low-sodium broth of choice or cold filtered water

1 teaspoon white sesame seeds

½ teaspoon lemon juice

Sea salt and black pepper

Pinch chili flakes (optional)

Parmesan cheese, grated (optional)

Heat the oil in a large pan over medium heat. Add the garlic and cook for 3 minutes, until the garlic browns slightly.

Add the asparagus and brown on all sides, letting one side brown then turning over to the other side, 10 to 15 minutes.

Add the broth or water. Cover and let simmer until the liquid is evaporated, 5 to 7 minutes. You want to look for a bright green color.

Add the sesame seeds and lemon juice. Season with sea salt and black pepper and finish with chili flakes and grated Parmesan, if you like.

Prep time: 10 minutes   Cook time: 10 minutes

burdock kinpira

Kinpira is a Japanese cooking technique that creates deliciously glazed umami vegetables. It's the perfect way to serve very subtly bitter burdock root—a food that helps the liver do its work and stokes the "fire" of digestion, but that can confound even an accomplished home cook. Adding iodine-rich seaweed and Kidney-supportive sesame seeds elevate the good-for-you qualities. The closer you can get your burdock and carrot into tiny matchsticks, the better. (Hint: Google "how to julienne cut" to sharpen your knife skills.)

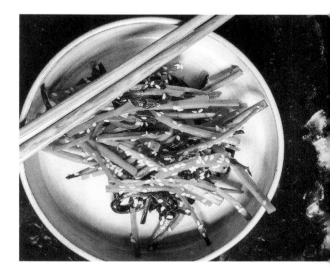

2 tablespoons avocado oil

2 cups (500 g) peeled, julienned burdock root

2 cups (500 g) peeled, julienned carrots

2 tablespoons hijiki seaweed, rehydrated in 1 cup (240 ml) cold filtered water, then drained

2 tablespoons pure sesame oil

2 tablespoons mirin

2 tablespoons tamari

1 tablespoon sesame seeds

Heat the avocado oil in a large sauté pan over medium-high heat. Once the oil begins to smoke, add the burdock, stirring to coat in the oil, and cook for 7 to 10 minutes, until the edges are browned. Reduce the heat to medium, add the carrots, and cook for another 5 minutes. Stir periodically, as the burdock tends to char quickly. Add the hijiki seaweed, sesame oil, mirin, and tamari. Stir to combine and then reduce the liquid until the vegetables are glazed, 5 to 7 minutes.

Sprinkle with the sesame seeds.

TIP Not sure about trying burdock? Let wise one Chad Cornell's words ring in your ears: "Good digestion leads to good circulation, which leads to good seed."

VEGETABLES

roasted spaghetti squash

SERVES 6

In the ramp-up to pregnancy, many women do well by reducing their carbohydrate load if it has fallen into excess. Swapping out boxed grain-based pasta—with its typically higher carbohydrate value—for a pasta-like vegetable can help. Eating sweet-tasting squash isn't just nutritionally healthy; it signals safety and comfort to the Spleen and helps you feel grounded and content. Top it with MotherBees Beef Bolognese (page 172), Broccoli Rabe and Moringa Pesto (page 192), or just grass-fed butter, Parmesan, and pepper.

1 spaghetti squash

1 tablespoon extra-virgin olive oil or avocado oil

Sea salt and black pepper

Preheat the oven to 350°F (175°C). Cut the spaghetti squash in half lengthwise and remove the seeds with a spoon. Season with the oil, sea salt, and black pepper and place the squash skin facing up on a parchment paper–lined sheet pan.

Bake for 30 to 45 minutes, until the squash is tender. Pierce the skin with a fork; if it punctures with no resistance, then it is ready. Take the squash out and flip it face up. Allow to cool for 20 minutes. Then, with a fork, scrape the squash away from the skin.

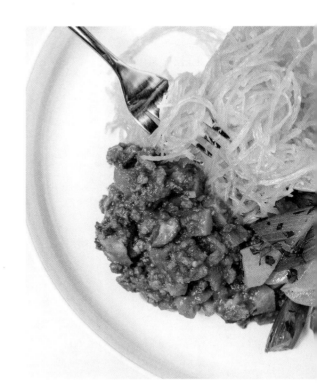

Prep time: 10 minutes   Cook time: 45 minutes

simply celery and carrots

SERVES 2

Perhaps the most humble vegetable dish ever, this uses two staple ingredients found in crisper drawers nationwide. Instead of making them the basis for soups, they're enjoyed in their own right: grounding, sweet carrots and restorative, alkalinizing celery are infused with broth, ghee, and garlic and topped with parsley to make a side dish that's so nurturing, it's made many a repeat appearance in a MotherBees bowl.

2 tablespoons grass-fed butter or ghee

½ clove garlic, thinly sliced

2 medium carrots, peeled, cut into 2-inch (5 cm) sticks at an angle

2 celery stalks, cut into 2-inch (5 cm) sticks at an angle

1 cup (240 ml) low-sodium broth of choice

Sea salt and black pepper

¼ cup (5 g) coarsely chopped parsley

Heat the butter in a large pan over medium heat, then add the garlic. Cook until the garlic begins to brown, then add the carrots and celery. Cook for 10 minutes, or until the edges start to brown.

Add the broth and cover. Simmer until the broth has evaporated and the vegetables are tender and ready to eat.

Season with sea salt and black pepper, then toss in chopped parsley at the end.

Prep time: 15 minutes   Cook time: 20 minutes

seasonal veggie succotash

SERVES 2

Succotash is a quintessentially American recipe. My inner artist relishes the quiet act of cutting all the vegetables the same size so the tiny cubes jumble together like colorful art. Eating succotash is like popping lots of daily multivitamins, every color infusing your body with nutrition and vitality. Get creative: if carrots, peas, green beans, or summer squash catch your eye, mix them in. Use what looks freshest and most energized with chi.

3 tablespoons extra-virgin olive oil

1 clove garlic, finely chopped

½ medium yellow onion, diced

1 medium red bell pepper, diced

1 medium zucchini, diced

1 cup (185 g) frozen lima beans

1 pint (300 g) cherry tomatoes, halved

¼ cup (5 g) chopped parsley

Sea salt and black pepper

Heat the olive oil in a large sauté pan over medium-high heat. Add the garlic and onion and cook until translucent, stirring constantly, for 5 to 7 minutes.

Add the red bell pepper, zucchini, lima beans, and cherry tomatoes. Cook over medium heat for another 10 to 15 minutes, until tender.

Finish with parsley and season with sea salt and black pepper to taste. Serve warm.

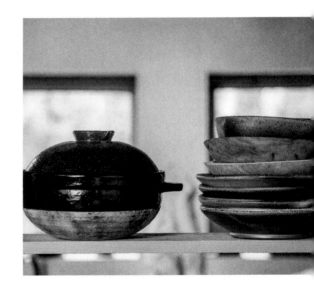

Prep time: 15 minutes   Cook time: 20 minutes

SAVORY SAUCES (AND ONE SWEET)

My terrific kitchen colleagues at MotherBees joke that "sauce is boss." Have a few tasty sauces in your kit, and you can make even the most mundane-seeming meal quite exciting. This quartet of simple sauces work with the Protein recipes and also will inspire you to drizzle, dip, and pour them on all kinds of basic bowls you already prepare for breakfast, lunch, or dinner. Each one offers ingredients that support your organ systems and help your hormone health—consider them sneaky ways to add more diversity and nutritional value to your plate.

cardamom ginger applesauce

Cooling apples and warming cardamom, nutmeg, and ghee combine in a sweet-tart sauce you can use to flavorfully accent pork dishes like the Pork and Kabocha Squash Stew (page 170), swirl into a simple congee or full-fat yogurt, or eat straight with a spoon. Apples are a tonic for the gallbladder, the source of the bile that helps to move toxins and used hormones out of your body. Made soft by cooking, they become extra nurturing.

1½ pounds (700 g) apples, peeled, cored, cut into medium cubes

1 (¼-inch/6 mm) knob fresh ginger

1 cup (240 ml) apple cider or apple juice

Juice of ½ lemon

½ teaspoon ground cardamom

Ground nutmeg

1 tablespoon ghee

In a medium pot over medium heat, combine the apples, ginger, apple cider, lemon juice, cardamom, and pinch of nutmeg and simmer gently so the apples soften properly before the liquid evaporates completely, 20 to 25 minutes. Poke an apple with a fork to see if it is tender. Once soft, turn off the heat.

Slowly pour the apples along with the ghee into a blender and blend until smooth.

Prep time: 15 minutes   Cook time: 25 minutes

nutty green yogurt sauce

SERVES 2

I created this sauce almost by accident, wanting to get selenium-rich Brazil nuts, mineral- and chi-rich herbs, and the all-important sour taste from yogurt into everyday meals. (Selenium is essential for thyroid health and supports strong sperm.) It turned out to be a happy accident, so addictive that I use it to enliven kitchari, grilled fish and chicken, and even bean-filled stews! If you tolerate dairy well, raw yogurt will make this even more fortifying.

2 tablespoons finely chopped fresh dill

2 tablespoons parsley leaves

2 tablespoons sliced chives

1 cup (30 g) dandelion greens or spinach

½ cup (75 g) raw Brazil nuts, chopped (option: soak overnight)

1½ cups (375 ml) full-fat dairy or almond yogurt

1 teaspoon ground cumin

1 tablespoon Dijon mustard

Juice of 1 lemon

Sea salt to taste

Place the dill, parsley, chives, greens, Brazil nuts, yogurt, cumin, Dijon mustard, and lemon juice in a blender. Blend on medium-high speed for a few quick seconds, until everything turns smooth. Add a little water if needed.

Season with sea salt to your liking.

Prep time: 10 minutes   Cook time: 0 minutes

tartar sauce
SERVES 2

Homemade tartar sauce is the ticket if you've got Oyster Fritters (page 174) in the pan. This dip is your opportunity to lavish that fritter with hormone-balancing fats! Don't be fearful of mayonnaise—there are plenty of healthier varieties made with avocado oils or expeller-pressed oils, or you can whip it up yourself with extra-virgin olive oil. A pasteurized egg and fermented pickle add extra nutrient value. It's equally good on crab cakes or, why not, some DIY fish sticks!

1 cup (240 ml) cold filtered water

1 whole egg

¼ yellow onion, finely diced

¼ cup (40 g) finely diced lacto-fermented sweet pickle

Pinch sea salt

¼ teaspoon freshly ground black pepper

1 cup (240 ml) mayonnaise or Vegenaise

Juice of ½ lemon

2 tablespoons finely chopped parsley

1 teaspoon whole-grain mustard

Pour the cold water into a small pot and gently place the egg in it. Over medium-high heat, bring the water to a hard boil. As soon as the water boils, turn off the heat and cover. Set a timer for 10 minutes.

Once the timer goes off, pour out the hot water and place the egg in an ice bath (a small bowl with ice cubes and cold water). When the egg is cooled completely, remove the shell and mash the egg into small pieces with a fork.

Stir in the onion, pickle, sea salt, black pepper, mayonnaise, lemon juice, parsley, and whole-grain mustard.

Prep time: 15 minutes   Cook time: 10 minutes

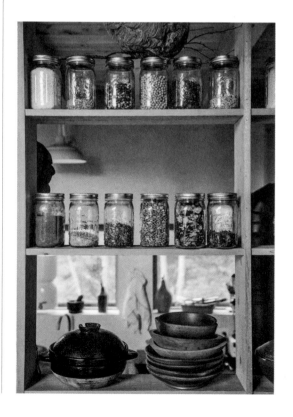

broccoli rabe and moringa pesto

SERVES 2

Ayurveda has long used the leaves of the moringa oleifera tree to treat a host of disharmonies. We now understand it's packed with vitamins and minerals, it's highly anti-inflammatory and liver-protective, and is rich with antioxidants that can protect eggs and sperm. Many use the leaf or powder as a tea, but get adventurous by integrating it into a pesto, and your lunch or dinner can become a fertility-protecting herbal tonic. (If you can't find moringa, use 2 cups/40 g arugula or spinach.) Pasta's the obvious contender, but I also like to dollop it on Kitchari (page 206).

2 cups (480 ml) cold filtered water, plus 2 tablespoons for blending if necessary

1 teaspoon sea salt

½ broccoli rabe bunch, ends cut off

½ cup (15 g) moringa leaves, all woody stems removed, leaves picked off, or ½ teaspoon moringa powder

1 clove garlic, finely chopped

¼ cup (35 g) raw almonds, soaked overnight in cold water filtered, peeled

Juice of 1 lemon

½ cup (120 ml) extra-virgin olive oil

Sea salt to taste

Bring the water to a boil in a medium pot over high heat and add the sea salt. Continue to boil, then add the broccoli rabe. Cook for 5 to 7 minutes, until tender. You are looking for a bright green color. Strain, then immediately place in an ice bath (a large bowl with ice cubes and cold water).

Once the broccoli rabe is cold, place in the blender with the moringa leaves (or powder), garlic, almonds, lemon juice, and olive oil and puree until smooth. If you are having a hard time getting all the ingredients to blend properly, you can add a couple of tablespoons of water to help the blades start to move again.

Season to taste with sea salt and let cool.

TIP Fresh moringa leaves can be found at some Asian markets and even at some farmers' markets. Moringa powder is easily sourced online and can be used in smoothies, too. A little powder goes a long way!

Prep time: 10 minutes   Cook time: 5 minutes

BROTHS, SOUPS, AND STEWS

Getting in the rhythm of making broth and soup weekly is one of the most powerful steps in feeding your preconception body well. If homemade broths with subtle medicinal touches are ready to go in your fridge or freezer, you always have the basics on hand to quickly replenish yourself between meals or make a heartier soup. If vegetables are cooked and pureed into gem-toned soups, there's no way around it; you'll drink them up daily, filling your reserves.

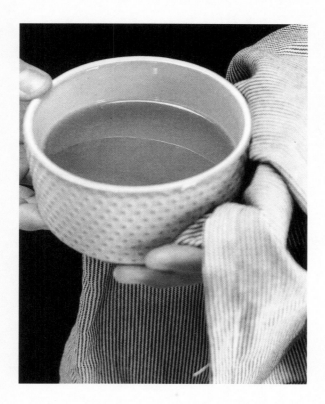

silken chicken broth

Traditionally, silken chicken broth is a prized food given to new mothers during the Chinese tradition of *zuo yuezi* or "sitting the month," because it delivers serious fortification to a body in need of recovery. Yet let's rewind: a woman's preconception body can be vulnerable, too, requiring extra replenishment and care. This exotic-sounding yet simple-to-make clear broth can help circulation, nourish the Liver and Kidney, invigorate the Spleen, and replenish chi. He shou wu is a root that has powerful antioxidant properties, builds the blood, and preserves jing.

1 whole silken chicken (or black chicken)

10 cups (2.4 L) cold filtered water

1 (2-inch/5 cm) knob ginger, thinly sliced

1 carrot, cut into 2-inch (5 cm) pieces

1 celery stalk, cut into 2-inch (5 cm) pieces

5 whole red dates (dried jujube), pitted

6 dried longan berries

¼ cup he shou wu root slices (optional)

Sea salt

Rinse the chicken inside and out and cut into 4 large pieces, leaving the head and feet attached. Set aside on a plate.

Boil the water in a medium pot over high heat. Add the silken chicken, ginger, carrot, celery, red dates, longan berries, and he shou wu, if using. Reduce the heat to medium-low and continue to cook for up to 1½ hours. Maintain 2 inches (5 cm) of liquid over the chicken.

Once cooked, let the mixture cool. Then strain, discarding the meat. (It is edible but typically not eaten.) Season the broth with sea salt to taste and warm up when ready to serve.

TIP Silken or black chicken is a specialty item found fresh or frozen in Asian markets, and even at some online retailers. It has a delicate flavor, slightly medicinal, in fact. It might take a foodie adventure to find it—my hope is you might enjoy the hunt! It's smaller than regular chicken and traditionally the meat is not used. If you can't find it, you can adapt this recipe to a regular chicken broth.

BROTHS, SOUPS, AND STEWS

Prep time: 30 minutes   Cook time: 1½ hours

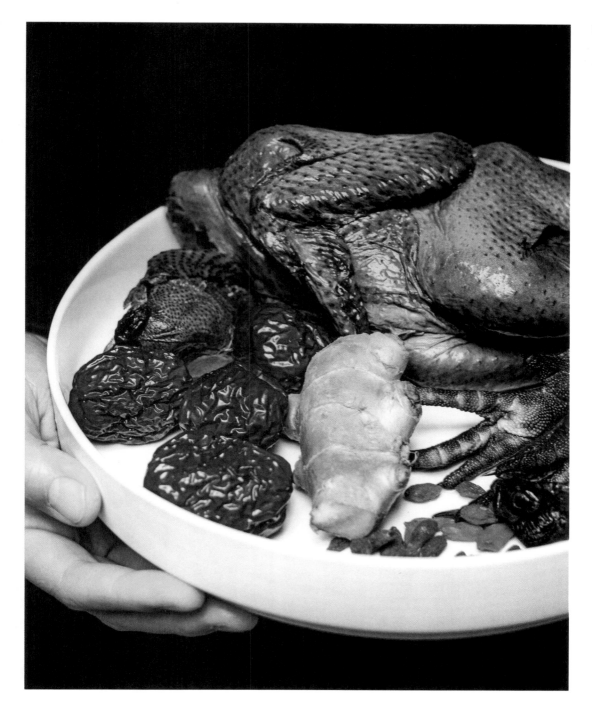

replenishing red soup

SERVES 4

It's not just green soup that's good to have on tap—ruby-red soup made from liver-boosting and blood-building beets is another plant-based tonic I recommend making every week. The iron and folate in beets are beneficial to both parents-to-be, and their nitric oxide increases circulation and healthy blood flow. Humble beets help your uterine lining replenish. You might especially appreciate this toward the end of your cycle. Added bonus? It's cheaper and more warming than costly beet juice from a juice bar.

2 large red beets, peeled, cut into ½-inch (12 mm) cubes, beet greens chopped and reserved

2 carrots, peeled, cut into ½-inch (12 mm) cubes

2 celery stalks, cut into ½-inch (12 mm) cubes

4 dried shiitake mushrooms

10 cups (2.4 L) cold filtered water or broth of choice

1½ teaspoons apple cider vinegar

1 teaspoon coconut oil

Sea salt and black pepper

Nutritional yeast powder

1 tablespoon plain full-fat yogurt or Nutty Green Yogurt Sauce (page 190) per serving

In a medium pot, combine the cubed beets, carrots, celery, mushrooms, and water or broth. Bring to a boil, then reduce to a slow simmer and cook for 20 to 30 minutes, until the vegetables are tender.

In two batches, transfer the soup to the blender, add the apple cider vinegar, and blend until smooth.

Heat the coconut oil in a small sauté pan over medium-high heat and sauté the beet greens until they wilt and have a nice caramelized look.

Season the soup to taste with sea salt and black pepper, nutritional yeast, and a dollop of yogurt or Nutty Green Yogurt Sauce, topping with the beet greens.

Prep time: 30 minutes   Cook time: 30 minutes

lentil soup with greens and grains

SERVES 4

This plant-rich soup deeply nourishes the three yin organs that support your reproductive potential. The lentil, legume, and quinoa proteins and the walnuts build up your Kidneys, the dandelion supports your Liver, and the warming, soupy quality nurtures your Spleen. It's also high in fiber, which your body needs to maintain hormone balance and which helps regulate blood sugar.

¼ cup (50 g) pearled barley

2 tablespoons coconut oil

2 carrots, diced

½ yellow onion, diced

2 celery stalks, diced

1 clove garlic, roughly chopped

¼ cup (30 g) raw walnut pieces, soaked overnight in cold filtered water

Pinch chili flakes (optional)

¼ cup (50 g) split red lentils

¼ cup (50 g) canned unsalted chickpeas, drained

¼ cup (45 g) white quinoa

8 cups (2 L) low-sodium veggie broth

1 cup (30 g) dandelion greens or spinach, cut into 2-inch (5 cm) strips

¼ cup (5 g) finely chopped parsley

Sea salt and black pepper

1 tablespoon nutritional yeast powder

In a small pot, bring 2 cups (480 ml) water to a boil and cook the barley over medium heat until tender, roughly 30 minutes. Drain and reserve.

Meanwhile, heat the coconut oil in a medium pot over medium heat. Add the carrots, onion, celery, and garlic and cook for 10 minutes, or until they begin to brown, stirring frequently.

Add the walnut pieces, chili flakes (if using), red lentils, chickpeas, white quinoa, and veggie broth and cook for 20 minutes.

Finally, add the cooked barley, dandelion greens, and parsley and simmer for 5 minutes.

Season to taste with sea salt and pepper, sprinkle with the nutritional yeast, stir, and enjoy.

TIP Lentils are full of magnesium and assist in the body's production of mood-boosting serotonin, helping to smooth out stress and tension. Try soaking and sprouting them to unlock their full vitality or chi—instructions for this are easy to source online.

BROTHS, SOUPS, AND STEWS

Prep time: 15 minutes   Cook time: 1 hour, 5 minutes

warming ginger cauliflower soup

SERVES 4

This super-easy blend of cauliflower, ginger, and coconut never makes it to the fridge—and for good reason. It tastes so creamy and nurturing, you barely realize you're helping to balance estrogen thanks to detoxifying compounds in the cauliflower, absorbing essential omega-3 fats and progesterone-supportive magnesium from the soaked walnuts, and enhancing circulation with the ginger. You can whip this up with barely a thought—if you're sharing it, just be ready for there to be no leftovers.

1 tablespoon coconut oil

½ cup (65 g) diced yellow onions

1 (1-inch/2.5 cm) knob fresh ginger, peeled, coarsely chopped

1 medium cauliflower, destemmed, cut into small florets

1 cup (115 g) raw walnut pieces, soaked overnight in cold filtered water

1 (13-ounce) can unsweetened coconut milk

10 cups (2.4 L) low-sodium veggie or chicken broth

Sea salt and black pepper

1 green onion, thinly sliced, for garnish

Heat the coconut oil in a medium pot over medium heat. Add the onions, ginger, and cauliflower florets and cook for 10 minutes, or until they turn slightly brown on the edges.

Remove half of the cauliflower florets and add the walnut pieces, coconut milk, and broth. Bring up the heat from medium-low and cook for another 20 minutes.

Pour the contents of the pot into the blender in two batches, blending each until smooth.

Season to taste with sea salt and pepper. Garnish with the green onion and the reserved cauliflower florets.

TIP Research shows that men who consume 2.5 ounces of walnuts per day see benefits in sperm quality, vitality, motility, and morphology (the size and shape of the swimmers). That's a heck of a lot of nuts! But traditionalists say even small amounts help strengthen the Kidney organ system, the source of his reproductive energy.

Prep time: 10 minutes   Cook time: 30 minutes

chicken broth with red date and goji berry

SERVES 6

This twist on one of the most popular soup recipes in *The First Forty Days* is my staple broth, served to women at all phases of their reproductive journey. In TCM, red foods are believed to support circulation, nourish the Liver, and reinforce warm yang energy. Jujubes or red dates also deliver vitamin C, while goji berries are high in protective antioxidants. These two medicinal fruits help to regulate the menstrual cycle, balance hormones, and unblock stagnant chi. Sip this as a warm beverage at any time of day or before a hearty meal.

Place the chicken backs, chicken feet, celery, onion, carrots, ginger, and red dates in a large pot. Add the water and bring to a high boil, then reduce the heat to a simmer. In the first hour, skim gray impurities off the top with a skimming ladle and discard.

After 2 hours, taste the broth—you are looking for a balance of chicken flavor and sweetness. Add the goji berries and simmer for another hour.

Strain and season with sea salt to taste. Reheat each serving when ready to drink.

4 pounds (1.8 kg) chicken back bones

1 pound (500 g) chicken feet

2 celery stalks, cut into 2-inch (5 cm) pieces

1 yellow onion, quartered

2 carrots, unpeeled, cut into 2-inch (5 cm) pieces

1 (2-inch/5 cm) knob fresh ginger, peeled, halved

5 whole red dates (dried jujube)

3 quarts (2.8 L) cold filtered water

¼ cup (40 g) goji berries

Sea salt

BROTHS, SOUPS, AND STEWS

Prep time: 20 minutes   Cook time: 3 hours

cleansing and fortifying green soup

SERVES 4

Having a large mason jar of green soup in the fridge is heaven for your preconception body (and your mate's—you both need this vitamin-and-mineral-rich elixir). Soup lets you drink your cleansing, fortifying greens—and I mean a *lot* of greens—in a warm, smooth, and soothing way, ensuring you truly get your fill. Once you get this simple method down, you can freestyle a little, using what's freshest or most appealing—green beans, chard, or avocado blended in to make the cashews' enriching texture even richer. Enjoy this several times a week.

In a medium pot, boil the water. Blanch the asparagus, zucchini, collards, strained cashews, cilantro, parsley, and spinach, then cook for 5 minutes over medium-high heat. Reduce the heat to a slow simmer and cook for another 10 minutes.

In two batches, transfer the soup to a blender and blend until smooth. Season the soup to taste with sea salt, add the coconut oil and nutritional yeast, and top with a dollop of plain yogurt or Nutty Green Yogurt Sauce.

8 cups (2 L) cold filtered water

4 spears asparagus, ends roughly cut

1 small zucchini, cut into ¼-inch (6 mm) cubes

1 cup (75 g) roughly chopped collard leaves

½ cup (60 g) raw cashews, soaked overnight in cold filtered water

½ cup (25 g) cilantro

½ cup (25 g) parsley

2 cups (60 g) spinach

Sea salt

1 tablespoon coconut oil

1 teaspoon nutritional yeast

Plain full-fat yogurt or Nutty Green Yogurt Sauce (page 190)

Prep time: 20 minutes   Cook time: 15 minutes

black sesame rice porridge

SERVES 2

When wise one Dr. Jay Lokhande taught us his traditional conception ceremony, I was mesmerized by the sound of the seven-day ritual of consuming nightly rice porridge. He called it an ojas-building food; so simple and pure it creates space for consciousness to flow. This adaptation of his recipe will beguile you at any time, whether for a gentle breakfast or late-night supper—perhaps you'll even enjoy it with your beloved in those precious days of your fertile window. Consume it slowly, noticing any relaxation or contentment you experience, a sensation of "I am satisfied." Dr. Jay says that's the perfect state from which to start the parenting adventure.

Soak the brown and sweet rice in a small pot with cold filtered water overnight, making sure there is 1 inch (2.5 cm) of water sitting on top of the rice. Strain and rinse the rice under cold water 3 to 4 times.

Add the milk to the pot of rice and bring to a boil. Cook for 30 to 45 minutes, gradually reducing the heat from a boil to a light simmer. Add more milk if needed.

Once the rice is soft, turn off the heat and add the coconut sugar, ghee, cardamom, and sliced almonds. Stir and enjoy.

Remember to soak rice for the next night.

¼ cup (50 g) organic brown basmati rice, soaked in cold filtered water overnight

¼ cup (50 g) sweet rice (if you don't have this, then add another ¼ cup/ 50 g basmati rice)

Cold filtered water

5 cups (1.2 L) full-fat cow, goat, coconut, oat, or almond milk, plus more if needed

½ teaspoon coconut sugar or jaggery

1 tablespoon ghee

½ teaspoon cardamom powder

Sliced almonds

BROTHS, SOUPS, AND STEWS

Prep time: 5 minutes   Cook time: 45 minutes

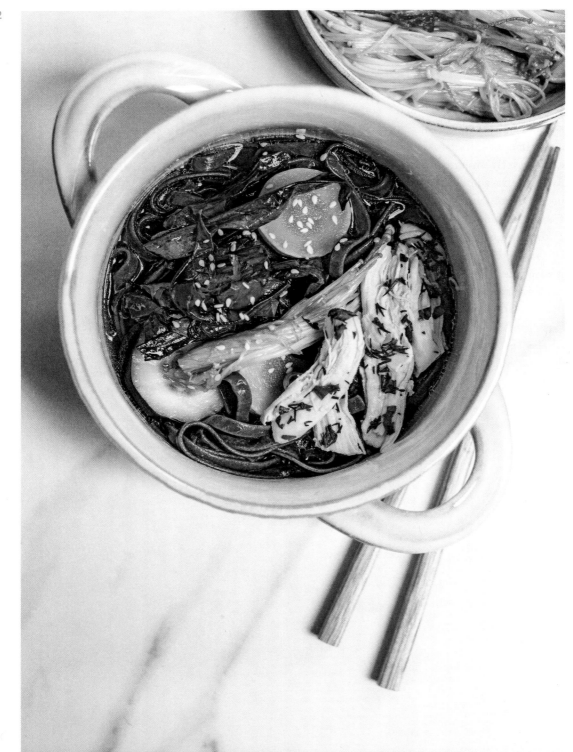

SERVES 2

When wise one Dr. Japa Khalsa described the Spleen/Stomach as the "inner child" who sometimes needs nurturing and comfort, I knew exactly why this easy chicken noodle soup hits the spot. It's so comforting! If you have broth ready to go in the fridge or freezer—one of the top preconception habits I advise—you can assemble this on even the busiest day. It's packed with fertility-protecting ingredients that burst with nutrition and vitality.

4 cups (960 ml) Chicken Broth with Red Date and Goji Berry (page 199)

1 boneless and skinless chicken breast

4 cups (960 ml) cold filtered water

¼ pack (2 ounces) black rice noodles (optional: Lotus Foods brand)

1 zucchini, skin on, sliced into ¼-inch (6 mm) rounds

1 pack (2.5 ounces) enoki mushrooms, destemmed, cut into 4 long bunches

1½ cups (45 g) dandelion greens or spinach, cut into 2-inch (5 cm) strips

2 tablespoons finely chopped parsley

2 tablespoons sunflower seeds

In a medium pot, heat the broth over medium heat. Bring to a light simmer, then add the chicken breast and cook for 10 minutes.

In a separate medium pot, bring the water to a boil and cook the brown rice noodles according to manufacturer's directions. Strain the cooked noodles under cold water and set aside.

After 10 minutes, take the chicken breast out of the pot and let it cool on a plate. Once the breast is chilled enough to the touch, shred the meat into strips using your fingers. Using the skimming ladle, skim any impurities off the top of the broth and discard.

Add the zucchini to the broth and cook for 5 minutes. Add the mushrooms and dandelion greens and cook for a final 4 minutes.

Place the cooked noodles and shredded chicken in a bowl and pour the broth on top.

Garnish with the chopped parsley and sunflower seeds.

Prep time: 15 minutes   Cook time: 30 minutes

BROTHS, SOUPS, AND STEWS

chicken mushroom congee

SERVES 4

If you haven't made congee by now, you haven't hung out with me long enough. Congee is my jam—it's a soft, warming, easy-to-digest rice porridge, a traditional Chinese dish that is often eaten in the morning to gently wake up the digestion. Once you locate sweet rice or "glutinous rice" (look for the Sho Chiku Bai brand), you can make this in a snap. This savory version includes a clutch of cleansing and fortifying foods including chicken liver—trust me, balanced with mushrooms and watercress, it will go down a treat.

¾ cup (155 g) jasmine rice

½ cup (100 g) sticky sweet rice

7 cups (1.7 L) chicken or vegetable broth

1 (1-inch/2.5 cm) knob fresh ginger, peeled, thinly sliced

2 tablespoons extra-virgin olive oil or avocado oil

1 pack (2.5 ounces) enoki mushrooms or oyster mushrooms, destemmed, split into 4 long bunches

1 bunch watercress

1 tablespoon grass-fed butter or ghee

2 pieces (40 g total) organic chicken liver, cleaned, coarsely chopped

Six-Flavor Chicken (page 178)

Soak the brown rice and sticky rice in a medium pot overnight with cold filtered water. The next day, wash and rinse the rice several times under running water until the water runs clear.

In the same medium pot, add the broth and ginger slices to the rice, then cook over medium heat for 30 minutes. Once the broth starts to bubble, reduce the heat to medium-low and let it simmer for another 30 minutes, maintaining 1 inch (2.5 cm) of liquid on top of the rice. Cook the congee for up to 1½ hours, stirring and adding water if the consistency gets too thick.

While the congee is cooking, heat a small sauté pan over medium heat, add the oil, and cook the mushrooms on both sides until they are lightly browned. Set aside on a plate. In the same sauté pan, sauté the watercress for 3 minutes over medium heat. Set aside.

Again, in the same sauté pan, heat the butter or ghee over medium-high heat. Add the chicken liver once the butter starts to smoke slightly. Once the liver starts to brown and the pink turns to a light brown, gently push down on the liver and check how firm it is. I tend to keep it slightly soft and not so tough to chew on.

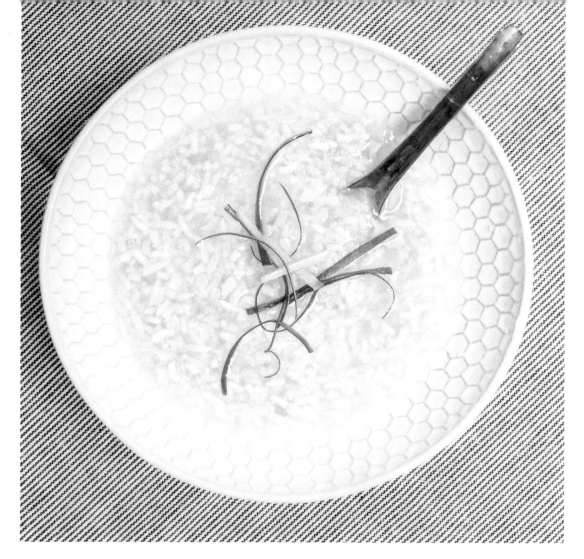

Once the congee is soft and thick, spoon a big heaping ladle into a bowl. Build your bowl with watercress, mushrooms, and liver, along with Six-Flavor Chicken.

TIP Once you've got your basic congee down, you can switch it up as you like, stirring in different ingredients like egg or vegetables, topping with other proteins, or swirling in black sesame seed paste. It can even become sweet—see *The First Forty Days* for some ideas!

Prep time: 15 minutes   Cook time: 1½ hours

kitchari with watercress and turmeric

SERVES 2

Kitchari is Ayurveda's trademark cleansing and rejuvenating dish. It's easy on the digestion, a sattvic food that creates peace in the body. I love inhaling the aromatic spices and adding handfuls of vegetables. Enjoy it on days you seek quiet; it's a wonderfully yin food.

3 tablespoons ghee

1 tablespoon whole fennel seeds

1 tablespoon whole cumin seeds

1 tablespoon whole brown mustard seeds

1 teaspoon ground fenugreek

½ teaspoon ground turmeric, or 1 small knob, fresh, grated

Sea salt and black pepper

1 (1-inch/2.5 cm) knob fresh ginger, peeled, finely chopped

1 medium carrot, peeled, minced

1 celery stalk, minced

½ cup (100 g) split red lentils

½ cup (100 g) organic brown rice, soaked in cold filtered water overnight

8 cups (2 L) vegetable broth

½ cup (65 g) sweet potato (peeled, cut into ½-inch/12 mm) cubes

½ cup (65 g) seasonal squash (cut into ¼-inch/6 mm cubes)

2 cups (60 g) baby spinach

1 cup (30 g) roughly chopped watercress

2 tablespoons raw almonds, soaked in cold filtered water overnight, peeled, chopped

Heat the ghee in a medium pot over medium heat, and when melted, add the fennel, cumin, and mustard seeds. Toast the seeds until you smell a nice aroma and the mustard seeds start to snap open. Add the fenugreek, turmeric, salt and pepper to taste, ginger, carrot, and celery, and cook, stirring, for 5 minutes.

Next add the lentils, brown rice (strain and rinsed a few times), and broth. Bring to a boil, then reduce the heat to medium-low to simmer, cover, and cook, stirring periodically, for 30 minutes.

After 30 minutes, add the sweet potato and squash, stirring, and cook for an additional 20 to 25 minutes, until the veggies and lentils are tender. You may need to add more broth if the kitchari gets too thick. You are aiming for the consistency of a stew (not too thick, not too thin).

In the last 5 minutes, stir in the spinach and watercress. Turn off the heat. Cover the pot and let it sit for 10 minutes.

Season to taste with sea salt and black pepper, then top with the chopped almonds.

Prep time: 20 minutes   Cook time: 2 hours

SWEET AND SAVORY SNACKS

At every stage of your mothering journey—from long before it begins to when you're really in the thick of it—please have nutritious snacks on hand. It's so easy to run yourself ragged and forget your body needs to eat. If you've crafted a few fun-to-eat munchables, packed with hormone-balancing and fertility-preserving ingredients, you'll help your energy and your cycle to stay on even keel and won't be tempted to grab the plastic-wrapped snack laced with who-knows-what. (And when children come into the picture, you'll be a well-prepared parent, homemade snack packs at the ready!)

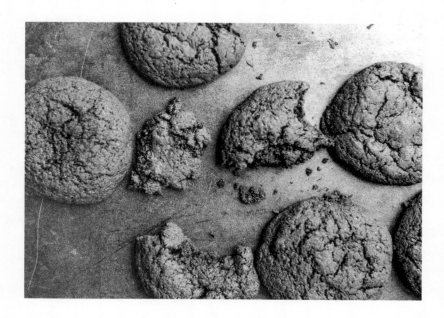

satiating chickpea crunch

SERVES 2

When you get a craving for a pop of crunchy, salty, snacky goodness, don't reach for a bag of chips! Try this twist on an Indian street food—your Kidneys will love the umami taste from the salt and nutritional yeast and your eyes will delight in the unexpected color from the spirulina, a blue-green, mineral-rich algae known to be one of the most concentrated whole foods on earth. While chickpeas have a ton of benefits, I don't suggest eating chickpeas daily; their phytoestrogens may work against fertility when consumed in abundance.

1 (15-ounce) can organic chickpeas, no salt added	½ teaspoon pure Hawaiian spirulina powder
2 tablespoons coconut oil	½ cup (25 g) nutritional yeast
Pinch sea salt	Juice of ½ lemon

Preheat the oven to 400°F (205°C). Open the can of chickpeas, strain over the sink, and run under cold water to rinse the chickpeas of canning brine. Place the strained chickpeas on a sheet pan lined with paper towels to try to remove as much excess water as possible, as this will help with crisping. Once the chickpeas are mostly dry, place them in a mixing bowl, add the coconut oil and sea salt, and mix.

Place the chickpeas back on the sheet pan and place in the preheated oven. Roast for 15 to 20 minutes, shaking the pan halfway through. The chickpeas are ready when they are slightly darker, crispy, and you will notice some have popped. At this point, remove them from the oven and place them back in the bowl.

Toss immediately with the spirulina, nutritional yeast, and lemon juice.

Let them cool for a bit to crisp up more, then enjoy.

TIP Spirulina comes from the sea; when picking a brand, read up on their sourcing to be sure it's safe and uncontaminated. Spirulina is a health powerfood partly because it helps the body eliminate metals. It should never be used when pregnant and not used in abundance in the weeks before you hope to conceive.

Prep time: 10 minutes   Cook time: 20 minutes

chili lime pepitas

SERVES 2

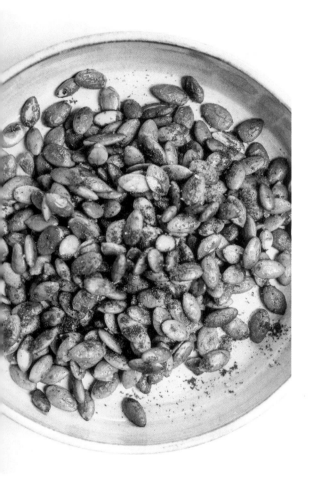

In TCM, seeds have a jing-like quality—they are the source of new life. Pumpkin seeds are especially great for preconception, high in magnesium and immune-boosting zinc, which is especially important for building healthy sperm. This Mexican twist makes them zesty and addicting. Scatter them on your green soup for an added kick of crunch and heat.

3 tablespoons avocado oil

2 cups (240 g) raw pumpkin seeds

Juice of ½ lime

1 teaspoon ground cayenne pepper

Sea salt

Heat the avocado oil in a medium sauté pan over medium-high heat. Once the oil is hot, add the pumpkin seeds to begin to toast. Make sure you are tossing and stirring them constantly as they begin to swell, toast, and pop, for roughly 10 minutes.

Once they are evenly toasted, turn off the heat, add the lime juice, and season with cayenne pepper and sea salt.

SWEET AND SAVORY SNACKS

salted almond date bites

MAKES 12 TO 14 BALLS

Ayurveda describes sumptuous, divine dates as a veritable ojas-building food. I love combining them with an array of hormone-balancing seeds including black sesame, a Kidney and Liver tonic my aunt used to spread on apples as a snack. These sweet and savory bites are an especially supportive snack during the follicular phase of your cycle (days 1 to 14). With the mixing and hand-rolling, making them can be a calming stress-release practice.

½ cup (40 g) coconut flakes

2 tablespoons black sesame seeds

12 whole, medium Medjool dates, halved, pits removed

1 tablespoon coconut oil

5 tablespoons (40 g) pumpkin seeds

1 teaspoon flaxseed powder

1½ tablespoons almond butter

2 tablespoons chia seeds

½ teaspoon pink salt

Prepare a food processor with the large S-blade attachment for mixing and blending. In a small bowl, set aside ¼ cup (20 g) of the coconut flakes and the black sesame seeds for rolling the balls.

Combine the Medjool dates, coconut oil, pumpkin seeds, flaxseed powder, almond butter, chia seeds, pink salt, and the remaining ¼ cup (20 g) coconut flakes in the food processor. Process on high for 5 minutes, or until the consistency is smooth and sticky.

With clean palms, create 1-inch (2.5 cm) balls of the mixture and roll in the coconut–black sesame mixture.

Keep refrigerated in a sealed container for up to 5 days.

Prep time: 20 minutes   Cook time: 0 minutes

coconut rose bites

MAKES 12 TO 14 BALLS

Rose is a famously heart-opening flower. Enjoy these fragrant bites with your lover or when you are feeling love for yourself (they can be an uplifting support while practicing any of the techniques in Clearing). The combination of sunflower and sesame seeds also supports the progesterone-rich stage of your cycle (days 15 to 28). Ashwagandha, an ancient medicinal herb, helps to reduce your cortisol levels and also boosts fertility in men—think of these as boosting virility, fertility, and romance.

½ cup (40 g) small coconut flakes

2 tablespoons rose water

12 whole, medium Medjool dates, halved, pits removed

1½ tablespoons sunflower butter

1 tablespoon coconut oil

1 tablespoon sunflower seeds

1 tablespoon white sesame seeds

½ teaspoon maca powder

½ teaspoon ashwagandha powder

1 teaspoon sea salt

Prepare a food processor with the large S-blade attachment for mixing and blending. In a small bowl, set aside ¼ cup (20 g) of the coconut flakes and the rose water for rolling the balls.

Combine the Medjool dates, sunflower butter, coconut oil, sunflower seeds, white sesame seeds, maca powder, ashwagandha powder, sea salt, and the remaining ¼ cup (20 g) coconut flakes in the food processor. Process on high for 5 minutes, or until the consistency is smooth and sticky.

With clean palms, create 1-inch (2.5 cm) balls of the mixture and roll in the coconut–rosewater mixture.

Keep refrigerated in a sealed container for up to 5 days.

Prep time: 20 minutes   Cook time: 0 minutes

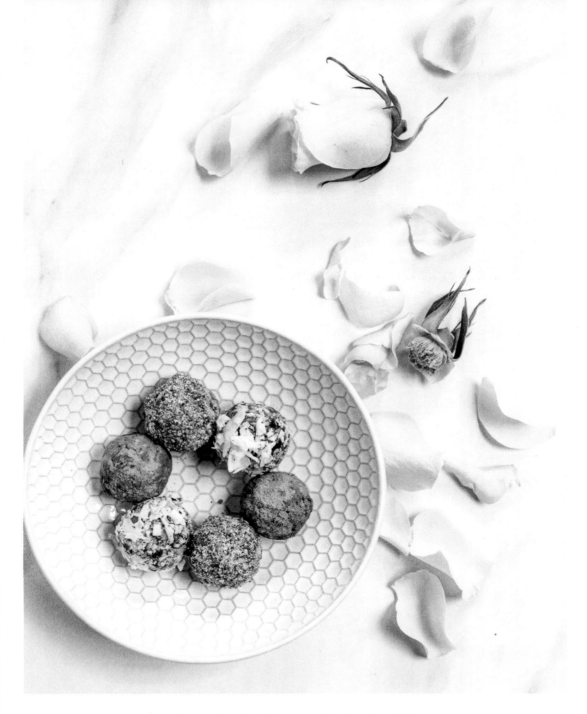

Clockwise from Top: Salted Almond Date Bites (page 210),
Coconut Rose Bites (page 211), and Apricot Turmeric Bites (page 213).

apricot turmeric bites

MAKES 12 TO 14 BALLS

These uplifting bites may be just what you need as your period concludes. Apricots and hemp seeds provide needed energy and ginger and turmeric help to reduce the inflammation that can naturally occur at the end of your cycle. But don't wait until the bleeding stops to indulge! They can be enjoyed whenever you need a tasty boost.

½ cup (40 g) coconut flakes

1 teaspoon turmeric powder

12 dried apricots, halved

1 teaspoon goji berries

1 (¼-inch/6 mm) knob fresh ginger, peeled

1 (¼-inch/6 mm) knob fresh turmeric, peeled

1 tablespoon coconut oil

¼ cup (40 g) shelled hemp seeds

2 tablespoons almond butter

½ teaspoon cinnamon powder

¼ teaspoon sea salt

Prepare a food processor with the large S-blade attachment for mixing and blending. In a small bowl, set aside ¼ cup (20 g) of the coconut flakes and the turmeric powder for rolling the balls.

Combine the dried apricots, goji berries, fresh ginger, fresh turmeric, coconut oil, hemp seeds, almond butter, cinnamon powder, sea salt, and the remaining ¼ cup (20 g) coconut flakes in the food processor. Process on high for 5 minutes, or until the consistency is smooth and sticky.

With clean palms, create 1-inch (2.5 cm) balls of the mixture and roll in the coconut–turmeric mixture.

Keep refrigerated in a sealed container for up to 5 days.

Prep time: 20 minutes   Cook time: 0 minutes

figgy chia pudding

This milky pudding is a treat for your eyes and senses, not just your reproductive center. In traditional medicines, visual similarity matters—certain foods help encourage certain functions, by virtue of their appearance. With their abundance of tiny seeds, figs and chia seeds help to encourage the profusion of healthy eggs and sperm. Figs, also a treasured ojas-building food, are high in fertility-supportive iron, zinc, calcium, and fiber. More than anything, this sensual treat will create pleasure through and through.

Once the pudding is set and is neither too liquid nor too thick, spoon into mason jars and garnish with the remaining ingredients.

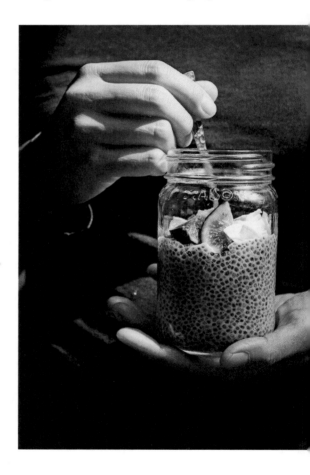

¾ cup (130 g) black chia seeds

½ teaspoon vanilla extract

4 cups (960 ml) full-fat, plant, or nut milk

2 tablespoons maple syrup

4 fresh or dried figs, quartered lengthwise

4 tablespoons (30 g) pistachios, chopped

4 tablespoons (25 g) coconut chips

Whisk together the chia seeds, vanilla extract, milk, and maple syrup. Place in the fridge for at least 2 hours, covered with plastic wrap, stirring periodically.

Prep time: 2 hours   Cook time: 0 minutes

blackstrap molasses cookies

MAKES 18 TO 24 COOKIES
(DEPENDING ON SIZE)

Blood-building blackstrap molasses contains all the vitamins and minerals that were absorbed by the sugar cane plant from the soil but don't make it through the refinement process of white sugar. With a robust flavor, these molasses treats are loaded with iron, antioxidants, and anti-inflammatory properties, and fragrant with warming cinnamon notes.

3 cups (410 g) whole-wheat flour

1 teaspoon baking soda

1 (2-inch/5 cm) knob fresh ginger, peeled, grated

1½ teaspoons cinnamon powder

1 teaspoon ground cloves

1 cup (225 g) raw salted butter

½ cup (175 ml) raw honey

½ cup (85 g) brown sugar

2 eggs

½ cup (165 g) blackstrap molasses

Preheat the oven to 375°F (190°C).

Mix the whole-wheat flour, baking soda, ginger, cinnamon, ground cloves, butter, honey, brown sugar, eggs, and blackstrap molasses in a large bowl.

With clean palms roll 1-inch (2.5 cm) balls and place 2 inches (5 cm) apart on a baking sheet lined with parchment paper. Bake for 6 minutes on the top rack, then move to the bottom rack and bake for another 6 minutes, until the top layer is firm to the touch.

Move to a cooling rack.

SWEET AND SAVORY SNACKS

Prep time: 5 minutes   Cook time: 12 minutes

NOURISHING MILKS AND HERBAL TEAS

Since my earliest days making food for mothers, I've loved serving milks. Warm, creamy, soothing concoctions that are rich in supportive fats, spiked with warming spices, and often laced with balancing herbs, they make a woman at any stage of her mothering journey feel cared for and complete. These variations use ingredients that especially support you and your partner during your preconception period. Enjoy them at the end of a long day or to take on the go with you so you never get depleted.

And make time for tea. Should you see a trained herbalist for support on your fertility journey, you and your partner would likely receive individualized instructions of herbs, tonics, and teas to address your needs for balance. Yet there are universal herbs that have a general tonic effect for reproduction, helping to balance hormones, regulate menstrual cycles, support sperm production in men, and prepare your body for pregnancy and childbirth. When you make them, you tap into the plant world's extraordinary repository of healing and fortifying compounds and start to become your own healer. You likely won't have them all at hand in your pantry, but they're easy to source online. (My favorite resource is MountainRoseHerbs.com.) Let them be the beginning of your own wise woman herbal medicine collection.

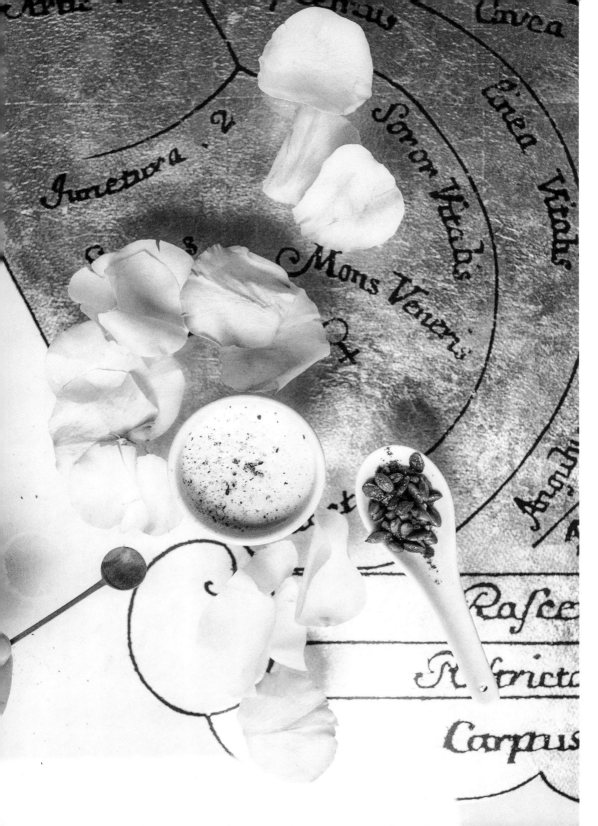

pumpkin seed and black sesame milk

SERVES 2

This milk is a fertility power trio, combining three building and balancing ingredients in one fortifying mug. Black sesame seeds are a tonic in TCM and Ayurveda, used to support menstrual cycle balance, fertility, and sperm health among many other things. They're also high in essential minerals.

2 cups (240 g) raw pumpkin seeds

1 cup (140 g) black sesame seeds

¼ cup (40 g) goji berries

4 cups (960 ml) cold filtered water

¼ teaspoon vanilla extract

In a sealed container, soak the pumpkin seeds, black sesame seeds, and goji berries in the cold filtered water and place in the fridge overnight. Make sure the seeds and berries are covered in water and there is about 2 inches (5 cm) of water on top.

In the morning, strain the mixture and put the mixture into a blender. Blend along with the cold filtered water on high for 2 minutes or until smooth.

Strain the mixture through a nut-milk bag into a mixing bowl. Gently squeeze the remaining liquid through the bag, making sure all of the liquid has been filtered through.

Stir in the vanilla extract and sip immediately.

Prep time: 10 minutes, plus overnight soaking

Cook time: 0 minutes

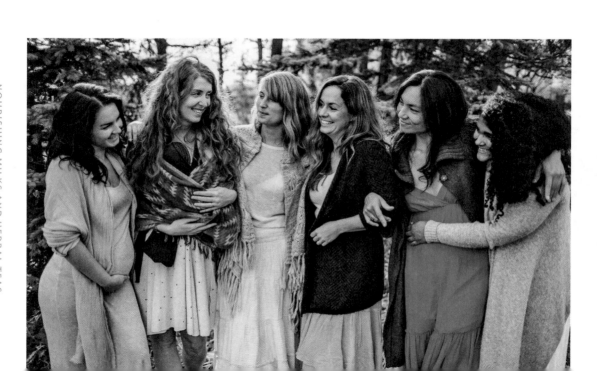

jing chai "life force" milk

SERVES 2

This milk is the motherlode of jing- and ojas-supportive ingredients—red dates, spices, ginger, and honey infused into warm, rich milk. Turmeric calms inflammation and supports the liver; reishi strengthens immunity; ashwagandha helps balance hormones. Let yourself sink into a state of relaxation as you take time to care for yourself—offer your partner a mug, too, and enjoy taking care of each other.

4 cups (960 ml) full-fat milk or organic almond milk

1 (1-inch/2.5 cm) knob fresh ginger, grated

3 red dates (dried jujube), pitted, finely chopped

½ teaspoon cinnamon powder

½ teaspoon cardamom powder

¼ teaspoon ashwagandha powder (optional)

¼ teaspoon reishi powder (optional)

½ teaspoon honey (optional)

Heat the milk in a small pot over medium heat then add the fresh grated ginger, red dates, and cinnamon and cardamom powders. Bring to a medium-low boil, then reduce to a light simmer and cook for 10 minutes.

Turn off the heat, stir in the ashwagandha and reishi, if using, and steep for another 10 minutes. Strain, add the honey, if using, and serve warm.

TIP Ashwagandha and reishi are an added boost. Even without them this blend will still be delicious, soothing, calming, and warming.

Prep time: 5 minutes   Cook time: 10 minutes, plus 10 minutes steeping

nettle and honey milk

SERVES 2

Nettle tea is a classic fertility tonic and a staple herb at MotherBees. This time-honored herb delivers essential nutrients like calcium and magnesium, tones the uterus and strengthens the adrenals, and infuses detoxifying chlorophyll into your body. For preconception, this super-creamy milk takes the benefits further, enriching nettles with the fat-soluble vitamins and essential fatty acids from raw dairy. If you can't find that near you, plant-based milks will work, just not quite with the same intensely building real-food effect.

3½ cups (840 ml) cold filtered water

2 cups (120 g) fresh nettles or 1 cup (45 g) dried nettle leaves

1 tablespoon raw honey

¼ cup (60 ml) raw milk

¼ cup (60 ml) raw heavy cream, or almond, oat, or coconut milk

1 tablespoon raw butter

recipe continues

In a small pot, boil the water over medium-high heat. Add the nettles and cover. Turn off heat after 5 minutes. Steep for 20 minutes over no heat.

Mix in the raw honey, strain, then add the milk, cream, and butter. Stir, and sip away.

TIP When spring hits I know nettles will start popping up through to early summer, easy to find at farmers' markets and also in my own backyard! It's a sign to get my tongs, kitchen knife, and kitchen mittens out. Once they are dropped into hot boiling water the stingers will fall off, and you won't feel them or taste them.

Prep time: 5 minutes
Cook time: 5 minutes, plus 20 minutes steeping

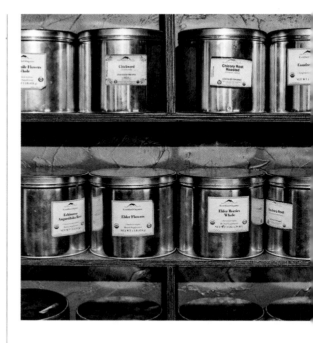

calming cinnamon eggnog

SERVES 1

This ovum-nourishing, nerve-calming elixir is a favorite of fertility expert Danica Thornberry and an ideal tonic for today's depleting, fast-paced world. The ginger adds a protective element to the raw egg—even so, use the best-quality egg you can find, ideally pasture-raised. This recipe is designed for those who can easily digest full-fat cow or goat milk (organic, if possible).

1 cup (240 ml) full-fat milk (options: kefir, raw, unpasteurized milk, or organic whole milk)

1 raw organic egg, yolk only

½ teaspoon raw honey

1 (¼-inch/6 mm) knob fresh ginger, peeled

½ teaspoon cinnamon powder

¼ teaspoon ashwagandha powder (optional)

Add the milk, egg yolk, honey, ginger, cinnamon powder, and ashwagandha powder (if using) to a blender and blend for 5 seconds.

Pour into a mug and drink straightaway.

Prep time: 5 minutes   Cook time: 0 minutes

berries, roots, and roses tea

SERVES 2

In TCM, juicy red Schisandra or "fruit of five flavors" is said to calm the heart and quiet the spirit. True to its name, the garnet berries will also take your taste buds on a joyful ride with sour, salty, bitter, sweet, and pungent notes (I like to balance the burst of flavor with a trace of gentle rose). Antioxidant-rich goji berries join in to make this a true health tonic that balances the key organ systems and supports the fertility of men and women. Brew up a big batch and sip anytime during the pre-conception period (avoid drinking this tea while pregnant).

¼ cup (60 g) whole dried Schisandra berries, soaked overnight in cold filtered water

4 cups (960 ml) cold filtered water

1 tablespoon goji berries

1 tablespoon sliced astragalus root

1 (½-inch/12 mm) knob fresh ginger, peeled

1 teaspoon dried rose buds (optional)

1 teaspoon honey or coconut sugar

Strain the Schisandra berries and set aside.

In a small pot, bring the cold filtered water to a boil over high heat. Add the strained Schisandra berries, goji berries, astragalus root, and fresh ginger root, and then turn down the heat to low. Simmer covered for 20 minutes.

Turn off the heat and add the rose buds, if using, then simmer covered for another 5 minutes.

Strain, add the honey, and sip hot.

TIP It is not advised to use Schisandra berries during pregnancy.

Prep time: 5 minutes   Cook time: 25 minutes

balancing and detoxifying tea

SERVES 2

In this quartet of women's health herbs, motherwort supports the heart, calms anxiety, and, like raspberry leaf, is a uterine tonic. Milk thistle strengthens and renews the liver, helping to create hormonal balance. Shatavari, aka wild asparagus, translates as "She who has one hundred husbands!" It's an Ayurvedic adaptogenic herb that can help regulate the menstrual cycle, boost immune health, combat stress, and increase cervical mucus. It is thought to balance the pH of your vagina and positively influence the release of luteinizing hormone (LH), necessary to help trigger ovulation. Shatavari is also great for breastfeeding and for use from perimenopause to menopause, as a natural

recipe continues

aphrodisiac, and is supportive for men's sexual function, too. If this blend tastes bitter to you, add a small amount of honey.

5 cups (1.2 L) cold filtered water

1 tablespoon motherwort leaves

1 tablespoon milk thistle leaves

1 tablespoon shatavari root

1 tablespoon raspberry leaves

1 tablespoon nettle leaves

1 tablespoon red clover blossoms

½ teaspoon honey (optional)

Bring the water to a boil in a medium pot over high heat.

Once the water boils, add all the tea leaves and roots. Reduce the heat to medium-low and simmer for 10 minutes. Turn off the heat, cover the pot, and let the tea steep for 20 minutes.

Strain the tea, add honey, if using, and sip away!

Prep time: 5 minutes   Cook time: 10 minutes, plus 20 minutes steeping

fertility tea for women and men

SERVES 2

Dong quai is known as the "women's herb" in TCM—it's sometimes referred to as "female ginseng" and is a classic blood tonic used once a young woman has begun menstruating. Yet it also aids male fertility, improving sperm motility, morphology, and count. Here it's paired with milk thistle and burdock root, bitter herbs that improve digestion, thus leading to stronger organs and healthier sperm and eggs. This unisex tea can especially support men on their preconception path, strengthening the whole package—sperm, mood, muscles, brain, courage, and self-esteem.

5 cups (1.2 L) cold filtered water

1 tablespoon ashwagandha root

1 tablespoon shatavari root

1 tablespoon dry burdock root

1 tablespoon milk thistle seed

1 teaspoon Chinese angelica (dong quai) root

½ teaspoon local honey (optional)

Bring the water to a boil in a medium-size pot over high heat. Once the water boils, add all the roots and seeds. Reduce the heat to medium-low and simmer for 10 minutes.

Turn off the heat, cover the pot, and let the tea steep for 20 minutes.

Strain the tea, add the honey, if using, stir, and sip while hot.

Prep time: 5 minutes   Cook time: 10 minutes, plus 20 minutes steeping

I dedicate this book to the calling within each woman that inspires her to create new life—or to create herself anew.

Awakening Fertility would not have been conceived without my team of superb, smart, and dedicated individuals who are now my dear friends. Special thanks to my coauthors, Amely Greeven and Marisa Belger, who spent countless hours researching, writing, and refining, all the while caring for their young ones; to my literary agent, Marc Gerald, and his wife, Cristina, who have always believed in my vision, and to my incredible editor, Holly Dolce, and the wonderful Abrams team for investing their faith and energy into this new book—a prequel to *The First Forty Days*.

The process of making this book was blessed by the creative talent of two übertalented photographers, Jenny McNulty and Elliana Allon; by my gifted book designer Laura Palese; by my wonderful MotherBees team member and research assistant Jennie Liu; and by our supportive recipe collaborators, Victor Boroda and Sara Martin. I will be ever grateful for the collective of wise women and men who shared knowledge from their life's work in order to inspire, empower, and comfort all who read these pages. And I honor my family, without whom this book would not exist—my elders who taught me and raised me, and my three beloved children who are the lights of my life: Khefri, India, and Jude.

May your journey to motherhood be filled with love, abundance, and acceptance for where you are along the path. ⬡

—HENG OU
(and in case you're wondering, it's pronounced "hahn oh") x

EDITOR: Holly Dolce
DESIGNER: Laura Palese
PRODUCTION MANAGER: Anet Sirna-Bruder

Library of Congress Control Number: 2019946926

ISBN: 978-1-4197-4384-9
eISBN: 978-1-68335-799-5

Abrams Image books are available at special discounts when
purchased in quantity for premiums and promotions as well as fundraising or
educational use. Special editions can also be created to specification.
For details, contact specialsales@abramsbooks.com or the address below.

Abrams Image® is a registered trademark of Harry N. Abrams, Inc.

ABRAMS The Art of Books
195 Broadway, New York, NY 10007
abramsbooks.com